D1002157

EARLY PRAISE FOR ABDUL EL-SAYED'S AND MICAH JOHNSON'S *MEDICARE FOR ALL*

"In this important and timely book, Drs. El-Sayed and Johnson document everything you need to know about Medicare for All. This Citizen's Guide both demystifies and humanizes our broken health care system and explains why we must fight to transform it now."

—Ady Barkan, Organizer, Center for Popular Democracy and Co-Founder, Be A Hero PAC

"Drs. El-Sayed and Johnson have written a lucid and accessible account of why Medicare for All is the best path for universal health care access in the US. Stripping the arguments 'for' or 'against' of sham ideological content, they make clear that the main question is whether we believe that no one should have to face both illness and financial ruin. If you agree, read this book to make the case!"

—Mary Bassett, MD, MPH, Director of the FXB Center at Harvard Chan School of Public Health and Former Health Commissioner, New York City

"This is by far the finest extended analysis I have seen to date of the next wave of public policy options for health care reform. It is breathtakingly comprehensive, thoroughly supported with research citations, lucidly written, and logical. It amounts to a major contribution to the US health care reform debate."

—Donald M. Berwick, MD, Former Administrator, Centers for Medicare and Medicaid Services

"Nurses have long understood that the major obstacle to passing Medicare for All isn't the policy, but the will to take on those who benefit from our immoral, profit-driven health care system. In this book, Drs. El-Sayed and Johnson brilliantly demonstrate how Medicare for All works, and how a combination of messaging and grassroots advocacy can overcome our opposition. A must read."

—Bonnie Castillo, RN, Executive Director, National Nurses United

"During a period when global pandemic has exposed the deadly mistake of linking health care to our workplace, *Medicare for All: A Citizen's Guide* is the sweeping, clear-eyed manual for making health care a right that we've been waiting for."

—Benjamin Day, Executive Director, Healthcare-NOW

"The growing debate over Medicare for All has mostly occurred at the level of soundbites and slogans, not specifics. In this essential 'Citizen's Guide,' we get the specifics: the provisions, promise, potential pitfalls of—and, yes, political prospects for—this bold vision for affordable quality care for all. Whether you support Medicare for All or just want to truly understand it, you must read this book."

—Jacob S. Hacker, Stanley B. Resor Professor of Political Science, Yale University and Author of *The Great Risk Shift: The New Economic Insecurity and the Decline of the American Dream*

"*Medicare for All: A Citizen's Guide* is part moving narrative, part detailed policy analysis, and part practical organizing playbook. . . . I am grateful to Drs. El-Sayed and Johnson for speaking truth to power in this fierce book."

—Representative Pramila Jayapal, WA-07

"This book is a labor of love for the American people and the health care system they deserve. Drs. El-Sayed and Johnson demystify Medicare for All and defang the political talking points to offer a clear distillation of the potential of this policy, while guiding the reader through the challenges and opportunities of this moment for achieving it."

—Representative Ro Khanna, CA-17

"In this timely book, Drs. El-Sayed and Johnson shine a light on the people left behind by our current health care system. Regardless of your politics, their thought-provoking writing will push you to think more deeply and critically about the future of health care in America."

—Vivek H. Murthy, MD, MBA, 19th Surgeon General of the US

"If the American health care system were a patient, it would be in critical condition. Fortunately for us, Drs. El-Sayed and Johnson don their white coats to discuss the diagnosis, prognosis, and therapeutic options in plain English. This incisive handbook is a must-read for anyone trying to make sense of one of the most pressing issues of our time."

—Danielle Ofri, MD, PhD, Clinical Professor of Medicine and Author of When *We Do Harm, A Doctor Confronts Medical Error*

"In this book, Drs. Abdul El-Sayed and Micah Johnson discuss Medicare for All in clear and simple terms. They describe the reasons why the industry has opposed the policy even though it would help millions of Americans, and how everyday Americans are beginning to make Medicare for All possible."

—Senator Bernie Sanders, VT

"The coronavirus pandemic has revealed just how unsustainable our fragmentary, privatized, and fundamentally individualistic health care system truly is. This engaging and accessible guide couldn't have come at a better time."

—Lindsay F. Wiley, JD, MPH, Professor of Law and Director of the Health Law and Policy Program, American University Washington College of Law

"An essential primer on why we need Medicare for All, the essentials of reform, and the pitfalls to avoid in crafting legislation."

—Steffie Woolhandler, MD, MPH, Distinguished Professor of Public Health, City University of New York and Co-founder of Physicians for a National Health Program

MEDICARE FOR ALL

ABDUL EL-SAYED AND MICAH JOHNSON

A CITIZEN'S GUIDE

OXFORD
UNIVERSITY PRESS

OXFORD
UNIVERSITY PRESS

Oxford University Press is a department of the University of Oxford. It furthers the University's objective of excellence in research, scholarship, and education by publishing worldwide. Oxford is a registered trade mark of Oxford University Press in the UK and certain other countries.

Published in the United States of America by Oxford University Press
198 Madison Avenue, New York, NY 10016, United States of America.

Library of Congress Cataloging-in-Publication Data
Names: El-Sayed, Abdul, author. | Johnson, Micah, author.
Title: Medicare for all : a citizen's guide / Abdul El-Sayed & Micah Johnson.
Description: New York, NY : Oxford University Press, [2021]
Identifiers: LCCN 2020020821 (print) | LCCN 2020020822 (ebook) |
ISBN 9780190056629 (hardback) | ISBN 9780190056643 (epub)
Subjects: LCSH: Medicare. | Medical care—United States. | Medical policy--United States. | Health care reform—United States.
Classification: LCC RA412.3 .E47 2021 (print) | LCC RA412.3 (ebook) |
DDC 368.4/2600973—dc23
LC record available at https://lccn.loc.gov/2020020821
LC ebook record available at https://lccn.loc.gov/2020020822

3 5 7 9 8 6 4 2

Printed by Sheridan Books, Inc., United States of America

Abdul: to Emmalee, my reminder of the future we must yet build.

Micah: to Cindy and Cliff, for a lifetime of inspiration and support.

The authors: to an America where healthcare is a right, not a privilege.

CONTENTS

FOREWORD BY SENATOR BERNIE SANDERS

During the greatest pandemic in modern American history, Americans suffered worse than our counterparts in other industrialized countries because we are the only ones who do not guarantee healthcare to every person as a human right. People went without the healthcare they needed. Hospitals were left on the brink of collapse when we needed them most—all because we have maintained an enormously dysfunctional, wasteful, and bureaucratic system that enriches the CEOs of the health insurance and pharmaceutical industry but leaves tens of millions of Americans without basic healthcare. This is shameful.

The fight for Medicare for All has been the fight of my life. Throughout my career, I have heard from Americans of all walks of life who have shared heartbreaking stories about our system. Older Americans have told me about having to ration their medications because of the outrageous price of prescription drugs. Doctors have told me about their patients who have died because they put off seeing a doctor because it was too expensive. Cancer patients have told me about suffering without the treatments they need because they are too expensive.

Even though more than 87 million Americans are uninsured and underinsured, we spend far more for healthcare per person than any other industrialized nation. Even though the Canadians, French, and British spend less than half of what we do, they have higher life expectancies and lower infant mortality rates than we do.

The solution, in my view, is simple. More than 50 years ago, our government established Medicare to guarantee the right to comprehensive health benefits for Americans over 65. It has been extremely successful, popular, and cost-effective. It is time for us to expand and improve Medicare to cover ALL Americans. That is why I introduced the Medicare for All Act into the U.S. Senate. Under this legislation, we would provide every American comprehensive coverage, saving money for middle-class and working families by eliminating the costs of their private insurance and replacing it with a publicly funded plan.

Some have said this would be too expensive. Others have said it's unworkable. Still others have said it would take away Americans' choice. These critics play on the fears of Americans and ignore the clear and simple truth of Medicare for All. It would make American healthcare more efficient, more affordable, and more reliable. It is why dozens of grassroots organizations, including the National Nurses United, have been such strong advocates for this plan.

In this book, Drs. Abdul El-Sayed and Micah Johnson lay out the facts about Medicare for All. They discuss the policy in clear and simple terms. And they describe the reasons why the industry has opposed our legislation even though it would help millions of Americans, and how everyday Americans are beginning to make Medicare for All possible.

I ran for president on a simple idea. Not me, Us. Medicare for All is about us—and the future we want for our children and grandchildren. Its time has come.

Senator Bernie Sanders
Washington, D.C.

FOREWORD BY REPRESENTATIVE PRAMILA JAYAPAL

Medicare for All: A Citizen's Guide was written during an unprecedented crisis.

As of November 2020, the COVID-19 pandemic had claimed more than 240,000 American lives, a striking number that is greater than the number of American lives lost during World War I. This public health crisis also triggered the worst economic crisis since the Great Depression, with more than 45 million workers filed for unemployment. And that mass unemployment crisis became a mass uninsured crisis—millions of people lost their healthcare simply because they lost their job, joining the 87 million people who were already uninsured or underinsured.

Next to the sheer devastation of massive numbers of deaths, the most striking injustice has been the tremendous racial disparities of COVID-19 deaths and illness. Black Americans have nearly five times the odds of being hospitalized as white Americans and are twice as likely to die from COVID-19.[1] In the midst of this emerging news

[1] Centers for Disease Control and Prevention, "COVID-19 Hospitalization and Death by Race/Ethnicity," https://www.cdc.gov/coronavirus/2019-ncov/covid-data/investigations-discovery/hospitalization-death-by-race-ethnicity.html.

came the deeply necessary and incredibly painful awakening of millions of Americans to the horrific legacy of white supremacy, racism, and anti-Blackness. As George Floyd cried to breathe, America had its reckoning with police brutality and institutionalized racism—not new, certainly, but brought to the forefront with the multiple crises that faced our country.

COVID-19 shed a light on problems that existed long before the pandemic, including the deep lack of healthcare that led to too many Americans with chronic health conditions that had been unable to access care. Nearly half of all adults under the age of 65 were uninsured or underinsured even before the first American tested positive for COVID-19. Black Americans, Latinos, and Indigenous people are much more likely to be uninsured. For many of these individuals, COVID-19 threatened not only serious illness, but bankruptcy.[2]

And while, prior to COVID, arguments kept being made for how Medicare for All would destroy the "choice" that an employer-sponsored healthcare plan offers, no one made that argument after COVID hit. Then, tens of millions of Americans lost not only work but also their employer-sponsored insurance.[3] Now more than ever, we saw exactly how unsustainable it is to have a corrupt, for-profit healthcare system that ties insurance to employment.

[2] Commonwealth Fund, 2018 Biennial Health Insurance Survey.

[3] Steffie Woolhandler and David U. Himmelstein, "Intersecting US Epidemics: COVID-19 and Lack of Health Insurance," July 7, 2020, *Annals of Internal Medicine*.

It is a well-known fact that Americans pay more per capita for healthcare than any other country in the world, and yet healthcare in America—a patchwork of services with enormous gaping holes in coverage and cost, rather than a "system"—leaves millions without access to lifesaving treatments. This patchwork of services squeezes out billions of dollars in profits for health insurance companies, even as half a million Americans go bankrupt every single year because of medical bills.[4] We all know a story of a family member, friend, or colleague who has avoided getting the healthcare they need or filling a prescription because they couldn't afford it. In the richest country in the world, this is an outrage.

But all is not lost. There is a solution, a solution that has been tested and works in major countries around the world to guarantee healthcare to every person without premiums, unaffordable out-of-pocket expenses, and exorbitant prescription drug costs. It's a solution that includes reproductive healthcare, dental and vision, mental health, and long-term support services for our elderly and people with disabilities.

That solution is Medicare for All. It's a solution that simply cannot come quickly enough. Every second we wait is more lives lost.

I am the proud lead sponsor of the Medicare for All Act of 2019, which would guarantee comprehensive healthcare

[4] Himmelstein et al., "Medical Bankruptcy: Still Common Despite the Affordable Care Act," *American Journal of Public Health* 109, no. 3 (March 2019).

to all U.S. residents. As the Co-Chair of the Congressional Progressive Caucus and Co-founder of the Medicare for All Caucus, I have worked tirelessly with the Medicare for All movement that has swept our country. As the National Health Policy Chair for Senator Bernie Sanders's 2020 presidential campaign, it was an honor to work with outstanding champions like National Nurses United, Public Citizen, and the powerful Medicare for All grassroots movement to ensure healthcare is not a privilege for the few, but a human right for all. And it has been a true honor to work closely with Dr. Abdul El-Sayed and Dr. Micah Johnson in the fight for a more just and sustainable healthcare system.

In their book, Dr. El-Sayed and Dr. Johnson diagnose the problems in our healthcare system and make a compelling case for why Medicare for All is the way forward. Combining the best of journalistic storytelling and academic rigor, they outline with clarity and passion exactly how Medicare for All could work to cover all Americans while saving money. They break down complex policy questions with nuance, walking the reader through what a Medicare for All transition would look like, what the alternatives to Medicare for All are, and how we can create a political movement that finally makes Medicare for All the law of the land.

Medicare for All: A Citizen's Guide is part moving narrative, part detailed policy analysis, and part practical organizing playbook. Whether you are a patient, policy wonk, politician, passionate organizer, or curious citizen, you will gain knowledge, understanding of the challenges and the opportunities before us, and the need for every American to take a stand to fight for healthcare—as a human right for everyone, not a privilege for the wealthiest few.

This book is a fantastic contribution to our growing movement. In the span of a few short years, over half of the Democratic caucus has co-sponsored the Medicare for All Act of 2019. For the first time, we've had historic hearings in Congress speaking to the need and feasibility of Medicare for All. We have earned the support of grassroots organizations, unions, and voters. And new polling shows most Americans support Medicare for All.[5] We have more and more candidates for Congress running unapologetically on Medicare for All and winning—even in swing districts across the country. Thanks to organizers, policymakers, citizens, union members, activists, and patients across the country who have formed the bedrock of this movement, we have moved Medicare for All squarely into the political mainstream—so much so that we have unleashed a flood of millions of dollars from insurance and pharmaceutical companies to fight our movement.

So—we have much more to do to win this urgent battle. That work rests on the need for more Americans to fully understand what Medicare for All is, how it works, and how it will help everyone to live healthier lives where insulin treatments, cancer treatments, or basic day-to-day

[5] Public Opinion on Single-Payer, National Health Plans, and Expanding Access to Medicare Coverage; Poll: 69 percent of voters support Medicare for All.

prescription drugs will never again be unaffordable. Never again will an American have to wonder if they must choose between paying for their necessary healthcare or paying their rent.

Dr. El-Sayed and Dr. Johnson provide us with what we need to move forward and build our movement even stronger. We know we have tough days ahead of us. We know that no progress in this country, from Social Security to unemployment insurance to racial justice, has come without a mass movement from the grassroots and a real fight from established interests. And we know that we cannot stop fighting until all Americans, regardless of race, income, disability, documentation status, sexuality, or gender identity can access the healthcare they need and deserve.

I am grateful to Drs. El-Sayed and Johnson for speaking truth to power in this fierce book and for being in this fight with us. Join us: together, we can organize, demand healthcare as a right, and achieve real change in this country.

Congresswoman Pramila Jayapal
Washington, D.C.

ACKNOWLEDGMENTS

We are indebted to the many people who helped make this book possible. We're grateful to the team at Oxford University Press for seeing the potential in this book and helping bring it into being. They include our editor Sarah Humphreville as well as Emma Hodgdon and Amy Whitmer. We're also grateful to Chad Zimmerman who helped us conceive of the book in its earliest stages.

We thank Lisa Cardillo for generously sharing her time and her story. The work also benefited from a number of interviews with veterans of the healthcare debate in the US, including Dr. David Himmelstein, Dr. Don Berwick, Dr. John McDonough, Melinda St. Louis, Rep. Pramila Jayapal, Rep. Ro Khanna, Prof. Sherry Glied, Dr. Steffie Woolhandler, and several former government officials whom we interviewed off the record.

We benefited from the critical reads of Adrianna McIntyre, Ben Wilcox, Dr. Cliff Johnson, Dr. Dave Chokshi, Dr. David Himmelstein, Dr. Don Berwick, Dr. Jonathan E. Fried, Dr. Khin-Kyemon Aung, Michael Lighty, Dr. Rahul Nayak, Sib Mahapatra, Dr. Steffie Woolhandler, Dr. Stephanie Kang, Suhas Gondi, Prof. Ted Marmor, and Dr. Zirui Song. We appreciate the excellent research support from Emiliano Valle and Vincent Lin. This work would not have been possible without the diligent care and support of Tara Terpstra, as well as the hustle of Austin Fisher.

We are also grateful for our experiences in policy and politics that have informed our perspectives on the issues in this book. Abdul ran for Governor of Michigan on a platform of single-payer healthcare, campaigned as a surrogate for Sen. Bernie Sanders during the 2020 Democratic presidential primary, was appointed by Sen. Sanders to the Biden-Sanders Unity Task Force on Healthcare, sat on the 2020 Democratic National Committee Platform Committee, and campaigned as a surrogate for Vice President Joe Biden and Sen. Kamala Harris during the 2020 presidential general election. Micah was a lead author on the single-payer plan proposed by Abdul during his run for Governor, served as a health policy fellow in the U.S. House of Representatives in the office of Rep. Lloyd Doggett, provided technical assistance to Sen. Elizabeth Warren's presidential campaign, advised members of the Biden-Sanders Unity Task Force on Healthcare, and served as a policy volunteer for the Biden-Harris campaign during the 2020 presidential general election. We thank everyone who has shared their expertise and mentorship along the way. The views expressed in this book remain ours alone.

Abdul is deeply grateful for Dr. Sarah Jukaku's never-ending patience and support—as well as the constant joy and inspiration from Emmalee El-Sayed.

Micah extends his deepest thanks to Cindy, Cliff, Jacob, Hannah, Sam, and Libby.

MEDICARE FOR ALL

INTRODUCTION

The genius of the American experiment is that it set out to establish a nation founded on the will of the people. That aspiration is framed best in the U.S. Constitution, a prescient document whose preamble sets out a series of intents for a new system of government.

One of those intents is to "promote the general welfare." We've long struggled to meet the aspirations framed in that document, but this one is particularly challenging. Although it's difficult to get an accurate assessment of what the state of the general welfare was when those words were written in 1787, it's safe to say it was far worse than it is now.

Best estimates suggest that life expectancy for white men was thirty-eight years.[1] Such figures were sparsely recorded for women, who lacked all but the most basic rights in that time. They also leave out the nearly 700,000 Black Americans living in the United States, over 90 percent of whom were enslaved.[2] The inhumane circumstances of their lives mean that death and disease were certainly far more common among them, and even today their descendants continue to suffer from a life expectancy that is nearly four years shorter.[3]

We're tempted to think that with a life expectancy of thirty-eight, people just dropped dead in the prime of life. But in fact, life expectancy is an average, dragged down by deaths in infancy and early childhood. In 1787, nearly one in five babies died before their first birthday. Another one in five died before the age of five.[4]

That's largely because the germ theory of disease was still a century in the future, and the era of modern medicine that it ushered in was even further away. The most common causes of death were all infectious diseases—pneumonia, tuberculosis, cholera, dysentery, and smallpox. These infections have a predilection for the young, whose immune systems aren't yet fully developed. Without modern vaccines or antibiotics, what little medicine was practiced was done at home. Surgeries, from minor tooth extraction to limb amputation, were performed without anesthesia—and without sterile equipment. Much of it was deadly. None of it was particularly effective.

And yet as early as 1798, the Fifth Congress passed—and President John Adams signed—an early attempt by the fledgling republic to promote the general welfare, An Act for the Relief of Sick and Disabled Seamen.[5] At that time, international trade was vital to the well-being of the United States, although being a sailor was a particularly dangerous trade. To protect its merchant marine, Congress passed the law creating a system of government-run hospitals for seamen, funded by a mandatory tax on their earnings.

As science advanced through the nineteenth and twentieth centuries, American government acted as a catalyst to convert new knowledge into broad improvements in general welfare: improving sanitation, putting fluoride in drinking water, ensuring widespread vaccination, funding new hospital construction, and guaranteeing health insurance for senior citizens. Modern healthcare has developed tools that humanity couldn't have imagined in 1787, from vaccines and antibiotics to robotic surgery and targeted immunotherapy. Because of these advances and so many others, nearly 250 years after the people of the United States ordained and established the Constitution, American life expectancy has more than doubled.

And yet perhaps by the standards of our time—and the power and wealth of our country—we are yet failing to promote the general welfare. Life expectancy in the United States is nearly six years shorter than in Japan, the longest-lived country in the world. American infant mortality ranks fifty-fifth in the world. And American health disparities by race and socioeconomic status are among the world's steepest. Perhaps worse, life expectancy has stagnated, even *falling* for three straight years between 2015 and 2017.[6] Rather than the infectious diseases of the past, the diseases with a predilection for the young today are *diseases of despair*—drug overdose, alcohol misuse, and death by suicide. For the population at large, cancer and heart disease are the top killers.

For this mediocrity, Americans pay by far the steepest price for healthcare in the world. We spend 18 percent of all of the money in our economy on healthcare. We are projected to spend over $12,000 per person on healthcare in 2021, double the average in comparable countries.[7] And our costs are increasing rapidly.

Those increases have fallen hardest on poor, working, and middle-income Americans. One in ten Americans have no healthcare coverage at all. Those who do are seeing their annual insurance premiums explode, even as that insurance comes with rising deductibles and out-of-pocket costs that leave families financially and medically insecure. Indeed, more than two in five Americans who received a cancer diagnosis depleted their life savings within two years.[8]

Americans mostly agree that our system ought to provide accessible, affordable, dependable, and equitable healthcare to all Americans. However, we differ dramatically on how to do that. Some prefer that government directly take up the cause laid out in the Constitution—to promote the general welfare. Some argue that healthcare is best left to the free market. Others sit somewhere in the middle.

This debate sits within a broader American conversation about how to best meet our individual and collective needs. The working consensus in our country is that the market should supply consumer goods like clothing, food, and entertainment, and government should supply collective goods like schools, fire services, and roads. Many of our political disagreements turn on where these lines should be drawn. The landslide election of Ronald Reagan in 1980 ushered in a new era of zeal for the privatization of everything from prisons to Medicare to public schools. With that era fading in the third decade of the twenty-first century, others are arguing that public responsibility for education should begin before kindergarten, or that public responsibility for health insurance should begin before the golden years.

Amidst this disagreement, one thing is certain: the idea that government has a role in meeting collective needs is neither new, nor radical, nor un-American. But there is a long history of claiming as much. When Social Security was being debated during the New Deal, Republicans in Congress cried that "the lash of the dictator" would descend upon the country, and that the plan would "enslave workers."[9] The American Medical Association first deployed the charge of "socialized medicine" to defeat a statewide health insurance proposal in California, Red-baiting the electorate into opposition. They enlisted a young Ronald Reagan, then an actor, to warn that Medicare would end American liberty as we knew it.

Yet Social Security and Medicare are among the most popular social programs in the history of the United States. Why the warnings that these laws would destroy the republic? Especially in health reform, ideological smears have long been used to disguise financial interests. Nearly since the advent of modern medicine, those on the business end of healthcare have framed the public debate in a way that helps guard their personal wealth. In the first half of the twentieth century, doctors—and especially the American Medical Association—were the leading practitioners of this strategy. With the rise of corporate healthcare in the late twentieth century, doctors passed the mantle to insurance companies, hospital conglomerates, and pharmaceutical companies to warn that while national health insurance might be a noble goal, in practice it would both wreak havoc on the American people and offend our most sacred values. The reward for blocking reform is maintaining a lucrative slice of the $4 trillion healthcare industry.

But the appetite for change is growing. Rising costs have led to declining health security, giving a fierce new urgency to the national debate about how to make our healthcare system work for everyone. Three words have dominated this new American debate: Medicare for All.

Medicare for All (M4A) is a simple idea: the government guarantees comprehensive health insurance to all Americans under a single, publicly funded plan. This is not a new idea—it was first proposed on the national scene as National Health Insurance by President Theodore Roosevelt. But it is an increasingly urgent idea, one that has grown in popularity and stature because of the urgency and scale of the challenges it is intended to meet.

Bursting back onto the scene during the 2016 presidential primary as championed by Senator Bernie Sanders, M4A has framed the debate—particularly in the Democratic Party—about healthcare in every major election since. And beyond healthcare, it has emerged as a major fault line regarding the very role government ought to play in American society.

Champions of M4A have sought to establish it as the answer to the urgent challenge posed by expensive and inaccessible healthcare. At the same time, it has threatened the power of a healthcare industry that controls nearly a fifth of our national GDP. Opponents have risen up to protect their stake in the American economy, framing the debate as one about choice and government intrusion upon American freedoms.

This political debate is the context in which most readers will come to this subject—bombarded by the imprecise and manipulative deployment of information intended to sway a vote. And in many ways, the political discourse about M4A has left us less informed but more passionate, because it is intended to sidestep our faculties of reason and target our emotions instead.

This book was written to do the opposite. We intend it to be an honest guide to the policy, politics, and potential of M4A. American healthcare is extraordinarily complex, and we hope you'll come away from this book with a deeper understanding of how it works. But the most important questions in health reform are not technical. They are questions about our values: who deserves healthcare, whether healthcare should be treated as a consumer product or a public good, how the costs of sickness should be shared.

These are questions for all of us, not just CEOs and lobbyists. However, too often complexity is used as an excuse to forestall change and lock people out of the conversation. We are writing this book to cut through the fog and lay bare what's really at stake in our healthcare debate.

Though this book is our best effort at an objective assessment of the policy, that is not to say we, as authors, are impartial. How could we be? Given the state of healthcare in America, our aspiration is to improve the system, not observe it dispassionately. Nevertheless, we come by our preferences honestly. Neither of us works for a for-profit healthcare corporation. We are young American doctors who have taken oaths to protect our patients, and we believe in our country's capacity to do better. It is that preference—for a healthier, more equitable America—that motivates this writing and our work. However, where we may be partial, we have opted for candor and transparency. This work also benefits from interviews with more than a dozen of the nation's leading experts in healthcare politics and policy we conducted for this book, and their perspectives have informed these pages as well.

In Part I of this book, we explore the healthcare system as it exists in America. We introduce you to Lisa Cardillo, whose brushes with the healthcare system typify the broader American experience. Using her experience, we diagnose the key problems in the system. We then explore the history of health reform efforts to illuminate how our current system came to be—and how it might be reformed in the future.

In Part II we examine M4A as a policy. We analyze how it works, mapped to the critical challenges of American healthcare established in the first part. We then explore the question of how it's paid for and consider the proposed alternatives to M4A.

In Part III we consider the politics of M4A. We trace the pathway, the strategy, and the tactics that will likely be deployed, as well as the key stakeholders in the coalitions for and against the policy. We also consider important swing constituencies, the policy levers that might move their support one way or the other, and the critical role of organizing. We close by exploring how all these forces will come together in the political arena.

We are grateful you are taking the time to read this book. Indeed, however urgently we are debating health reform today, there is no doubt that our Constitution, written all those years ago in 1787, predicated government by the people on the assumption that we would be an educated and engaged community of citizens. We hope this work will be a contribution to that end.

PART I

HEALTHCARE IN AMERICA

1
DIAGNOSIS

Lisa Cardillo will never forget her fifteenth wedding anniversary. After waving goodbye to their three children, Lisa and her husband, Dominic, drove across the state to Grandville, a few miles from Lake Michigan. They had more than their anniversary to celebrate: Dominic, who'd suffered a malignant brain tumor at just thirty-three years old, was three years past his cancer diagnosis. After a full year of treatment, including radiation, surgery, and chemotherapy, he was now down to a few MRIs a year to make sure that the cancer hadn't recurred. Eager for a fresh start, the Cardillos were excited for a weekend getaway filled with romantic sunsets, a brewery tour, and a Red Hot Chili Peppers concert.

But just as they were about to enjoy the day on Lake Michigan's sandy beaches, Lisa felt a sharp burning in the center of her chest. Then came the crippling nausea and abdominal pain. She'd read something on Facebook about a friend of a friend having similar symptoms a while back—a recollection that came rushing on now. Though Lisa was thirty-six years old and otherwise healthy, she knew that something was terribly wrong.

The Cardillos knew better than to call an ambulance—Dominic's had cost them $800 when he was first diagnosed. They rushed to the car and started Googling nearby hospitals. The nearest one was just twelve minutes away. Dominic stepped on the gas. Lisa's left arm started to go numb.

As Lisa walked into the emergency room, she went into cardiac arrest. With her heart no longer pumping blood, she crashed to the floor. The emergency room personnel started performing CPR then and there.

Over the next nine agonizing days at that hospital, Lisa was diagnosed with a heart attack caused by spontaneous coronary artery dissection—a deadly tearing of one of the arteries that supply blood to the heart. Though extremely rare, this condition has a predilection for young women, like Lisa. After her cardiac arrest, she went into heart failure. The doctors put Lisa in a medically induced coma and implanted a heart pump that would do the work that Lisa's ailing heart could not.

Thankfully, Lisa survived. But those nine days were only the beginning of her ordeal. She was discharged on a cocktail of cardiac drugs—some to manage the strain on her heart, some to reduce her blood pressure. For five months she had to wear a defibrillator vest.

All of this was extremely expensive. The hospital sent a bill for $185,460. The defibrillator vest was another $5,000 a month. Then more bills for cardiac rehab, follow-up appointments, and prescriptions.

Lisa was no stranger to medical costs. She'd learned more than she ever wanted to know about navigating insurance bureaucracies dealing with Dominic's treatment just a few years earlier. His twice-annual MRIs cost thousands of dollars, on top of the cost of his radiation, chemotherapy, and surgical treatment.

And the Cardillos have insurance. Unlike the 30 million Americans who don't have it, they have health coverage through Dominic's job as an automotive engineer. Before Dominic's diagnosis they had tried to save on premium costs by choosing an insurance plan with a high deductible, meaning they would need to spend more before insurance kicked in. That left them with $12,000 in uncovered medical bills for his care, which they were supposed to pay out of pocket. Owing ten different medical creditors money they didn't have, they quickly found themselves underwater. Though Lisa and Dominic resisted asking for help, their friends eventually started a GoFundMe page and threw an in-person fundraiser to partially allay their debts. Together, their friends and family raised nearly $8,000—just enough to get them back on solid footing. But when January 1 rolled around, their deductible reset and they found themselves back at square one paying for Dominic's ongoing treatment.

Beyond the financial toll, there was the personal toll. Lisa had spent hours on the phone with the various hospitals, clinics, labs, and imaging centers where they owed money—not to mention pleading with their insurance company to cover the costs of this or that treatment. More than once, she'd found herself crying to the faceless insurance bureaucrat on the other end of the line. "When your medical bills become more stressful than your husband's brain cancer diagnosis, something is not right," she told us.

After Dominic's diagnosis, they upgraded to a more expensive insurance plan: now their out-of-pocket costs were supposed to be capped at $7,000 per year. But there were also the unexpected costs they had thought their insurance would pay that it didn't. When Lisa had her defibrillator placed, for example, the insurance company said her anesthesiologist was out-of-network, meaning she'd have to pay an extra $1,500 out of pocket. Still recovering from her cardiac arrest, she was too tired to deal with it all. She tried to ignore the bills and convalesce before starting another round of fighting, cajoling, and even begging her insurers and creditors.

Medical calamity has forced the Cardillos to make decisions that they never imagined having to make. "Are we going to be able to take our kids on a vacation or are we going to pay these medical bills so they don't send us to collections? It's a balancing act, and it's something I never expected," Lisa said. They are constantly juggling their finances to meet the minimum payments for each of the creditors they've accumulated through their brushes with death.

Morbidly, Lisa jokes that her "favorite bill" is the one for "cardiopulmonary resuscitation"—the manual CPR she got in the emergency room. For $568, the hospital personnel saved her life. But because she hadn't met her deductible, she paid for it out of pocket. "It's the best $568 I ever spent," she said. But should she have had to spend it at all?

Lisa's heart condition is rare. But her experience with our healthcare system is not. Here's the truth: America is exceptional on virtually every healthcare measure. But more often than not, we're exceptional in exactly the *wrong* ways.

In a comprehensive study of the healthcare systems of eleven high-income countries, here's how America fared compared to our peer countries—places like Canada, Switzerland, and the United Kingdom.[1] We spend the most money on healthcare in the world—nearly twice as much per person than our peer countries on average. Our national healthcare bill in 2016 came to $9,400 per person, versus an average of $5,000 in our peer countries—and in 2021 we're projected to spend more than $12,000 per person.[2] For every dollar spent in our economy, 18 cents go to healthcare. The average in our peer countries is below 11 cents.

What are we getting for this money? The short answer: worse health. This starts from the first moments of life. American infants have the highest rates of death. A baby's chance of death is twice as high if his mom is Black instead of white.[3] American moms also die at the highest rates after giving birth. This discrepancy continues to the last moments of life: Americans die three years earlier than our peers abroad. It's no surprise we have the lowest satisfaction with our healthcare system among our peer countries—less than one in five Americans think our healthcare system works well.[4]

It gets worse. Even after the implementation of the Affordable Care Act (ACA), more than 30 million Americans still did not have health insurance in 2019.[5] Our peer countries have uninsured rates between 0 percent and 0.2 percent.[6] Ours is almost fifty times higher, at nearly 10 percent of the population. And Americans with insurance aren't getting the healthcare they need, either—more Americans report skipping medical care due to cost than in any other wealthy country. Those who do get the care they need are paying dearly for it. And if you're Black or poor, you're more likely to be on the wrong side of these statistics.

America is also the only advanced nation with a health insurance system that crumbled in the face of COVID-19. In most other countries, every single citizen kept their health coverage throughout the pandemic. In the United States, millions lost their health insurance along with their jobs as a deadly contagion spread all around them.[7] Many Americans—insured or not—were forced to avoid care for fear of the costs. And our hospitals and clinics were brought to the brink of financial collapse when private insurance revenue dried up.

America's healthcare system is in critical condition. In this chapter, we'll try to get to the bottom of the diagnosis.

First, let's review the basic anatomy of American healthcare. When it comes to health insurance, we have no unified system to get people covered. Instead, Americans are carved up into half a dozen different systems. First is employer-based insurance: about half of Americans have private insurance coverage through their job, like Lisa and Dominic Cardillo. Second is Medicare, a public insurance program operated by the federal government that mostly covers Americans over age sixty-five (along with Americans who have certain disabilities). Third is Medicaid, a public insurance program operated by the states that mostly covers low-income Americans. Fourth is individual private insurance, usually purchased through the ACA marketplaces by people who do not have other options for insurance. Fifth are other public programs like the Veterans Health Administration and the Indian Health Service. Sixth and finally, some 30 million Americans remain uninsured. Based on their insurance, each of these groups has different access to a combination of basic and advanced healthcare services: primary care, emergency room visits, dental care, hospitalizations, prescription drugs, surgery, and more.

Combining all these parts of the US healthcare system, in 2018 Americans spent a total of $3.6 trillion on healthcare.[8] Nearly three-quarters of that money goes to four places: hospitals, doctors' offices, prescription drugs, and insurance administration. A third of all spending—over $1 trillion a year—goes to hospitals. Twenty percent goes to doctors' offices. Ten to 15 percent is spent on prescription drugs, and 8 percent goes to the overhead costs of the insurance system. The rest is spread across smaller categories like nursing homes, dental care, home healthcare, ambulances, and public health.

Our healthcare costs are increasing rapidly. In 2021, US healthcare spending is expected to exceed $4 trillion. By 2025, it is projected to be over $5 trillion.[9]

Though our healthcare system is complex, its problems are clear. Let's break them down.

PROBLEM #1: OUR HEALTHCARE IS TOO EXPENSIVE

Our healthcare costs are almost double those in the rest of the world. Why is this?

Many people assume that our costs are higher simply because we use more healthcare. But that's not actually true. We go to the doctor *less* in America than people in nearly all of our peer countries—for comparison, Americans have an average of four physician visits per year, while Canadians have nearly eight. We also use hospitals less, in terms of both admissions and total days spent in the hospital.[10]

If we don't use more healthcare than other countries, how are we spending twice as much? The first reason is that our *prices* are higher for just about everything in healthcare, including hospital stays, doctors' visits, and prescription drugs. The second reason is that we spend far more money on healthcare administration than other countries do. These two cost drivers share an underlying cause: our insurance system, which both enables high prices and creates administrative complexity.

"It's the Prices, Stupid"

The first key driver of our high healthcare spending is embarrassingly simple: our prices are higher. Much, much higher. And much higher for just about *everything* in healthcare. A day in the hospital costs $5,220 in America and $765 in Australia.[11] A 30-day supply of Xarelto, a medication that prevents blood clots, costs $70 in the United Kingdom and $380 in the United States. The cost of delivering a baby is thousands of dollars higher in America than in Switzerland or South Africa. Hip replacements here are almost three times as expensive as in the United Kingdom. A CT scan of your belly costs $140 in the Netherlands and $1,100 here. An MRI in Switzerland is $310; here it's $1,430. Coronary bypass surgery in the United States costs over $78,000—twice as much as in Switzerland, and five times as much as in the Netherlands.[12]

In other words, American healthcare costs are high not because women like Lisa spend too many days in the hospital, or because men like Dominic get too many brain MRIs. Our costs are high because we're charged more for those same hospital days and MRI scans than people anywhere else on earth. For instance, in the summer of 2019 Dominic got a brain MRI for a total price of $940—a good deal by American standards. But if Dominic lived in the

United Kingdom, that scan might be priced at $450. In the Netherlands, it might be $200 or less.[13]

The title of a research paper by a group of influential economists sums up the first answer to why healthcare costs are so much higher in America: “It’s the prices, stupid.”[14] In this context, *price* refers to the total amount of money received by a hospital, physician, or drug company for providing a product or service. Depending on the service and the patient, some of the price might be covered by insurance and some of the price might be paid out of pocket by the patient. (Throughout this book we use “price” and “payment rate” interchangeably, referring to how much a healthcare provider receives for a service.)

American medical prices are the highest in the world. But they also vary in seemingly bizarre ways: within the very same hospital, the price of a service can double or triple simply based on what kind of insurance a patient has. Prices for Medicare patients are often closer to the international norm, but prices for privately insured patients are astonishingly high by global standards. Remember Dominic’s $940 brain MRI? If he was on Medicare, the price would have been less than $400.[15] Not quite the Dutch price, but lower than the British price. In more extreme cases, prices within the same hospital can be *ten times higher* for patients with private insurance compared to patients on Medicare—for the exact same service![16]

Why are prices so high for people with private insurance? To understand this puzzle we’ll focus on the example of hospital prices, because hospitals are the biggest source of healthcare spending in the United States and those prices are rising the fastest. Prices for physician services work similarly (though the problem is less severe), and later we'll tackle the unique causes of high drug prices.

Hospital prices in Medicare are lower than prices in private insurance for a very simple reason: negotiating power. Because Medicare is such a large program, it has the power to unilaterally set reimbursement rates for all the services it covers—and nearly every hospital in the country chooses to accept those rates. Hospitals simply don't have the leverage to demand higher prices from Medicare.

Private insurance works very differently. There are nearly a thousand health insurance companies throughout the United States, and each negotiates its own prices with hospitals.[17] A given insurance company might offer dozens of different health insurance plans, and each plan can have its own negotiated prices. Compared to Medicare, private insurance companies have very little leverage to prevent hospitals from increasing their prices.

Some people might assume that because most hospitals are nonprofit institutions, they wouldn't take advantage of their power to charge higher prices. But they do: hospitals raise prices year after year, and there's not much private insurance companies can do to stop it. Insurance companies can then pass these higher costs on to patients in the form of higher premiums and deductibles. For instance, from 2007 to 2014, hospitals raised their prices by 42 percent.[18] Over the same period, private insurance companies raised their premiums by 40 percent for families with employer-based coverage.[19] Deductibles nearly doubled.[20]

The US healthcare system simply does not have effective tools to prevent price increases in the private marketplace. Like so many Americans, Lisa and Dominic suffered the consequences: rising premiums, excessive deductibles, and huge charges for their care. Even though they had private insurance that was supposed to protect them if they got sick, they still found themselves burdened by debt because of the high price of healthcare.

The basic reason prices are so high is that private insurance companies simply lack the leverage to keep prices under control. But there are two additional forces that exacerbate this problem: hospital consolidation and a system of broken incentives for insurance companies.

Hospitals Have Become Local Monopolies

Healthcare is local. You can't ship healthcare, and it has to be nearby when you need it. That's why patients almost always seek care from doctors and hospitals in the geographic area where they live. It's why Lisa got her healthcare in Grandville, where she was on vacation, rather than near her home on the other side of Michigan.

When one or two hospitals dominate the local market, they have even more leverage to charge high prices to people with private insurance. That's exactly what's happening in the United States, and the problem is only getting worse. In

1990, two out of three hospital markets were highly concentrated. In 2016, 90 percent of hospital markets were highly concentrated.[21] The monopolization of the American hospital industry reflects a flurry of mergers, with hospitals buying up their competitors to enhance their own power. Throughout the mid-2000s, there were fifty or more hospital mergers every year. The Affordable Care Act accelerated provider consolidation, and since 2014 there have been over a hundred hospital mergers every year.[22]

The result is higher prices. That's because in the private market, prices are determined by the relative bargaining power of the two parties at the negotiating table. It's incredibly hard for an insurance company to say no to any demand from a hospital that has a monopoly on the local market—if an insurance plan doesn't cover services from that hospital, their product becomes essentially worthless to patients in that area.

Unsurprisingly, hospital prices in consolidated markets continue to increase every year. When hospitals merge in already concentrated markets, the price increases can be shockingly high, often exceeding 20 percent.[23] After Evanston-Northwestern Hospital bought Highland Park Hospital—essentially dominating the market on the North Shore of Chicago—in just a few years prices increased by a staggering 48 percent.[24]

We spend over $1 trillion every year on hospital care in the United States. It's no surprise that rising hospital prices are an important driver of our national health spending. These high prices get passed on to consumers in the form of higher premiums, lower benefits, and lower wages.[25]

Insurance Companies Keep Prices and Premiums High

Insurance companies do have at least one effective strategy for bringing down prices: buying up competitors to build monopoly power. Because prices depend on the relative bargaining power of insurers and providers, insurance companies are able to negotiate somewhat lower prices if they manage to dominate a market. For instance, consolidating from three companies to two companies in an insurance market is associated with a 5 percent drop in prices paid to providers.[26] Another study found that hospital prices in the most consolidated insurance markets were 12 percent lower than prices in the most competitive insurance markets.[27] (That's right: more competitive insurance markets had *higher* hospital prices.)

But there's a catch: when insurance companies consolidate and use their market power to negotiate lower hospital prices, they simply keep the savings for themselves. In fact, when insurers consolidate, premiums go up. For instance, a study of the Aetna-Prudential merger found that the consolidation was associated with a 7 percent rise in premiums.[28] This should come as no surprise: with less competition, insurance companies are more able to charge patients higher premiums.

In essence, consolidation allows insurance companies to squeeze both patients and providers—which is good for insurance company profits but leaves both consumers and providers worse off. This makes our private insurance market a lose-lose for consumers when it comes to controlling prices. A fragmented insurance market may lead to competition and lower premiums today—but weak insurers allow providers to charge increasingly higher prices over time, leading to cost growth and higher premiums in the long run. On the flip side, insurance market consolidation gives insurers more negotiating power to rein in the prices charged by providers—but this leads to low competition, so insurance companies can just pocket the savings as extra profits and raise premiums in the process.

Furthermore, even when insurance companies *could* negotiate lower prices, they often choose to keep prices high. Imagine a hospital and an insurance company sitting at the bargaining table. Hospitals obviously want high prices—that's their income. In theory, insurance companies should want to keep prices low—the less they pay to hospitals, the more they get to keep for themselves in profits. But the incentives don't always work this way. Paradoxically, insurance companies actually have incentives to keep prices *high* in many cases.

The first reason for this is that insurance companies are focused on fending off competitors. This means that an insurance company is actually willing to accept high prices from a hospital so long as the hospital promises to charge even higher prices to competing insurance companies. Contracts between hospitals and insurers often include this type of agreement—it's usually called a "most favored nation" clause, but we can call it a "most favored insurer" agreement. Take an example: Blue Cross Blue Shield (BCBS) is the dominant insurer in Michigan. In 2010, BCBS had "most favored insurer" agreements with the majority of hospitals in the state. In some cases, these contracts required hospitals to charge rival insurers up to 40 percent more.[29]

The hospitals win: they charge higher prices to everyone. BCBS wins: it keeps its dominant market share and makes it extremely difficult for potential competitors to enter the market. The lesson is that if you're an insurance company, high prices are okay if they let you maintain a pseudo-monopoly, which means you can charge high premiums and keep the profits. This is essentially collusion between big hospitals and big insurers to keep prices high—a classic market failure.

The second source of broken incentives is an unintended effect of policy. The ACA contained a provision that requires insurance companies to spend at least 80 percent of the premium dollars they collect on medical claims (or 85 percent for insurers selling to large employers). The intention of this "80/20 rule" was to put a cap on the acceptable level of insurance company administrative overhead and profit.

If you're an insurance company, what do you do? Keep the pie as large as possible. This means that insurers would rather charge high premiums and pay providers high prices, rather than keep premiums and prices low, because it means a higher profit for them. And if they fight too hard for lower prices, they'll violate the 80/20 rule and be forced to pay the savings back to consumers. Indeed, after the 80/20 rule was introduced, insurance companies did not decrease premiums—instead, they paid more to providers.[30] So in the end, the players we rely on to keep prices low are often incentivized to keep prices high.

Drug Prices Are Out of Control

The United States spends twice as much per person on prescription drugs than our peer countries. It's cheap to manufacture prescription drugs, often costing just pennies per pill. Drug prices are high because many of these pills are protected by patents, meaning that pharmaceutical companies can set the price as high as they want, and no other company is allowed to offer the product at a lower price.

Patents give drug companies and investors the incentive to put up large sums of money to research and develop new drugs. If they successfully bring a new drug to market, companies are rewarded with the right to charge high prices with no competitors for a specified number of years. However, this system can make drugs unaffordable for patients. Other countries navigate this tension by regulating the prices that drug companies are allowed to charge, or by negotiating as a country to get bulk discounts on new drugs.

The United States is different. We have virtually no regulations on how much pharmaceutical companies can charge for drugs, whether patented or generic. Profit-seeking companies know how to use this system to their advantage. As CEO of Turing Pharmaceuticals, Martin Shkreli bought an old anti-parasite drug frequently used by people with HIV. Overnight, he jacked up the price from $13.50 to $750.[31] He's not alone. As CEO of Mylan, Heather Bresch raised the price of EpiPens over 400 percent.[32] Politicians, the public, and the media skewered these CEOs for their unethical behavior. But at the end of the day, why did they raise the prices? Because they could.

Americans have very limited ability to negotiate for lower drug prices. Medicare is the largest purchaser of drugs in the United States, but by law, Medicare is *prohibited* from negotiating drug prices with pharmaceutical companies. (When Congress added prescription drug coverage to Medicare during the George W. Bush presidency, the pharmaceutical industry lobbied vociferously—and successfully—to ban Medicare from negotiating drug prices.) For their part, private insurance companies simply lack the negotiating power to secure drug prices anywhere near the international norm. In essence, drug prices are high because pharmaceutical companies have monopolies on their most lucrative products—and there's no countervailing force to keep prices in check.

Complexity Is Costly

Our private insurance system doesn't only enable high medical prices. It's also very costly in and of itself, saddling the American healthcare system with the highest administrative costs anywhere in the world.[33] High administrative spending is the second key reason that US healthcare costs are so high.

A comprehensive study estimated that in 2017, the United States spent $812 billion on healthcare bureaucracy—almost a quarter of the $3.5 trillion we spent on healthcare that year.[34] That's nearly $2,500 per person. Meanwhile, Canada's single-payer system spent only $550 per person on healthcare bureaucracy. For comparison, the $812 billion we spent administering the healthcare system in 2017 is larger than the budget for the US military, larger than the budget for the entire Medicare program, and more than we spend nationally on public K-12 education.

Both healthcare providers and insurance companies incur astonishingly high administrative expenses. As we'll see, the root cause of this spending is our fragmented system of private health insurance.

Doctors, hospitals, and other healthcare providers face an enormous administrative burden from our convoluted payment system. In total, American hospitals on average spend 25 percent of total revenues on administration—the highest in the world.[35] Physician practices employ an average of two administrative staffers for every three clinical personnel.[36] The toll on hospitals and providers comes to hundreds of billions of dollars every year.[37]

When journalists write about the administrative burden on providers, they often focus on the need to reduce "paperwork." It's true that administrative complexity means more forms to fill out, but the problem is more severe: Americans spend hundreds of billions of dollars every year supporting an *entire industry* of billers, coders, and other administrators whose purpose is to keep our byzantine payment system ticking along.

Beyond the stacks of paperwork, picture this: the Duke University hospital system has 957 beds and employs more than 1,500 billing clerks.[38] The Cleveland Clinic maintains over 3,000 insurance contracts, and each contract contains negotiated prices for over 70,000 services.[39] This means the Cleveland Clinic has *210 million* different prices for the services delivered in its facilities. It takes a lot of time and money to translate everything that happens in a hospital into one of these 210 million different prices—and then to communicate back and forth with the insurance company and the patient to figure out how everything is going to be paid for.

Researchers from Harvard Business School teamed up with researchers at Duke to find out exactly how much time and money was devoted to billing and coding in a health system, following individual medical bills from beginning to end.[40] They found that physicians and staff spent 73 minutes preparing bills for an average patient in the hospital. If the patient had surgery, physicians and staff spent 100 minutes preparing the bills. The emergency department in the study spent more than 25 percent of its professional revenue simply processing bills.

The researchers provided a clue as to why the administrative costs of the US healthcare system garner little attention: the administrators themselves are largely hidden from both patients and doctors. The billing organization was located in a 125,000-square-foot building more than ten miles away from the main academic campus, employing more than 1,500 full-time equivalent staff.

Insurance companies also spend hundreds of billions of dollars a year on their own administrative needs. On average, private insurers use 13 percent of premiums for administrative expenses and profit.[41] In contrast, the traditional Medicare plan has administrative costs between 2 and 3 percent.[42] This means that when we send our healthcare dollars to private companies rather than a public plan, we're surrendering 10 cents on every dollar to extra administrative needs and shareholder profits. In essence, we're paying a premium on our premium. In total, America spends nearly three times as much on insurance administration than our peer countries.[43]

Where does this administrative spending actually go? Some of it goes toward core activities that any insurer must perform, whether private or public: processing claims, monitoring for fraud, and so on. But Medicare shows that you can perform these core functions for just a couple of cents on the dollar. What about the rest? Some of it goes toward marketing budgets, which private companies use to compete with each other to attract enrollees (and often to target healthier customers). Some of it goes to pay multimillion-dollar corporate salaries. Some of it goes to pay commissions to the brokers who link up insurers with groups of customers. And so on. In short, there's no single place where this administrative spending is being unconscionably squandered. Rather, once we treat health insurance as a business, we accept the usual costs of doing business: aggressive marketing, layers of bureaucracy, competitive corporate salaries. Beyond these administrative needs, a sizeable chunk of insurance revenue is also kept as profit—for a large insurance company, this can range from 4 to 7 percent of total premiums in a typical year.[44]

It is inevitable that a healthcare system will spend some of its money on administration. But America is peculiar in its incredibly high levels. The root cause is our fragmented private insurance system—private insurers themselves require an extra 10 cents on every dollar to function as a business, and in turn the sheer number of insurance companies imposes a burden on providers that drains tremendous time and money away from patient care.

In summary, American healthcare is so expensive because we pay higher prices for hospital care, physician services, prescription drugs, and other medical care—and also because our administrative costs are the highest in the world. Our complex, fragmented insurance system permits these high prices while imposing an enormous administrative burden. *It's the prices and the administrative costs*—both of which are high because of how we pay for care.

Why Doesn't the "Free Market" Control Healthcare Costs?

Unlike other countries, the United States does not use government regulation to keep healthcare costs in check. But shouldn't the market be able to control healthcare costs, without government interference? Americans generally rely on market competition to improve products, reduce prices, and leave consumers better off, with low costs and high quality. If the free market was working in healthcare, Americans would be able to get excellent care at a low price, keeping our bodies and pocketbooks healthy. But we get the opposite: expensive care and the worst health outcomes in the developed world. Why isn't the market working in healthcare?

It's understandable why the market can't solve the problem of high administrative costs, since the private insurance market itself is the cause of administrative complexity. But why can't the market keep prices and other costs under control?

To answer this question, let's first consider what a well-functioning market looks like: consumers know exactly what they're buying, they face the full costs of their purchase, they have the time and ability to deliberate and make the most rational decision, they have many options for where (and from whom) they make their purchase, and they can choose to not make a purchase at all. A well-functioning market also has many buyers and many sellers, which means no single party has control over the prices—it's left to the "invisible hand" of the marketplace.

Healthcare violates every one of these principles.

Think about Lisa. When she started experiencing chest pain, she was worried she might be having a heart attack. But there's no way Lisa could have known that she was experiencing spontaneous coronary artery dissection, and there's no way she could have known what diagnostic tests and procedures she was supposed to "shop" for. Most of medicine works this way: we seek medical attention when we want to know what's happening to us and what we can do about it. That means we don't have the full information that's needed to shop around—which is one thing markets need to work.

If Lisa somehow knew what services she would ultimately need and was able to look up the prices of a cardiac catheterization and a mechanical heart pump, there's a further issue: because of insurance, she doesn't face the full cost of the care she "purchases." In a normal market, the price paid by the consumer is the same price that's received by the seller. In healthcare, insurance covers most of the costs of each service—another reason healthcare isn't like other markets.

More to the point, Lisa simply couldn't afford to use precious time to look up all the different places where she could go for care, research what services she might need and try to find their prices, cross-reference that information with the details of her insurance policy, and look up quality ratings and reviews to compare her different options. It is no exaggeration to say that if Lisa had spent time doing any of that after she felt chest pain, her heart probably would have stopped before she reached an emergency department—without any professionals around to resuscitate her.

Lisa also had no real alternative to "purchasing" the services she was provided. When she was on the operating table about to get the procedure that would save her life, she had no real ability to shop around, or to decide she didn't want to buy at all. Economists call this an "inelastic" demand, meaning it doesn't change, no matter the price. When you need lifesaving care, you'll pay whatever you're charged.

You might think that Lisa's case isn't representative because it was an emergency. But most of these same forces—missing information, insurance coverage, urgency, and lack of alternatives—are at play in the majority of healthcare decisions. Researchers at the Health Care Cost Institute estimate that at least 60 percent of healthcare spending goes toward these kinds of "non-shoppable" services. And even if up to 40 percent of healthcare spending is on theoretically "shoppable" services, insurance insulates patients from the majority of these costs—all told, a mere 7 percent of total healthcare costs come from out-of-pocket spending on shoppable services.

Even for healthcare services that are theoretically shoppable, the consolidation of our healthcare system introduces a further market failure: you can't shop around when your local market has been monopolized by a single health system. (Similarly, you can't shop around for a better deal on medication when the drug company has a patent-protected monopoly.)

Finally, even in the rare cases where all the conditions seem to be in place for patients to act like typical consumers, they simply don't shop around. Researchers tested this by looking at one of the closest things to a commodity you can find in healthcare: lower-limb MRI scans, which are abundantly available, often scheduled in advance, and have no meaningful difference in quality from one location to another. Patients in the study faced high out-of-pocket costs, giving them a financial incentive to shop around; they also had access to a price comparison tool. Even under these ideal conditions, patients simply did not price-shop: on average, patients bypassed six lower-priced MRIs between their home and the location where they received their scan.[45] Less than 1 percent of patients used the price comparison tool at all. When receiving healthcare, patients simply are not consumers in the traditional sense.

The upshot is that American healthcare prices are not determined by the "invisible hand" of a competitive marketplace. They're determined by powerful companies that take advantage of a broken market to keep prices high.

PROBLEM #2: TOO MANY AMERICANS CAN'T ACCESS HEALTHCARE

Even though we dedicate nearly a fifth of our economy to healthcare, Americans are not receiving the care they need. More Americans lack access to healthcare than citizens in any other wealthy country.

Most severely, as of 2019 more than 30 million Americans had no health insurance at all.[46] But even Americans with health insurance can face barriers that prevent them from accessing care. First, as detailed earlier, care is simply too expensive, even for people with insurance. Second, insurance often does not cover all the services Americans need. And finally, many Americans in low-income urban and rural communities simply don't have quality services available in their geographic area.

Too Many Americans Still Have No Health Insurance

Health insurance is the most basic way that people gain access to healthcare. But nearly 10 percent of the American population has no form of health insurance, including 7 percent of Asian Americans, 8 percent of white Americans, 11 percent of Black Americans, 19 percent of Hispanic Americans, and 22 percent of Native Americans.[47] To put it simply: as of 2021, healthcare is *not* treated as a human right in America.

Why are so many Americans uninsured? Nearly half of the uninsured report the cost of coverage is too high.[48] One in five said they lost coverage because they lost or changed jobs; 13 percent lost coverage because they earned too much money or otherwise were disqualified for Medicaid. Just 3 percent of the uninsured say they have no need for health coverage.

Who are the uninsured? About a third (more than 9 million) are eligible for ACA subsidies to help them buy insurance—but either they don't know they are eligible or the subsidized insurance is still too expensive. Almost a quarter of adults and children without insurance are eligible for Medicaid but aren't enrolled.[49] In practice, if these Americans were hospitalized, they would be enrolled in Medicaid at that time. The fear is that they are missing out on preventive and primary care—or even avoiding the emergency room when they're sick—because they're not aware that they are eligible for insurance through Medicaid. In that way, the fragmentation and complexity of our insurance system keep many Americans uninsured.

Furthermore, over 2 million Americans fall into the tragic "coverage gap": they're below the poverty line, but they don't qualify either for Medicaid or for subsidized insurance through the ACA.[50] This coverage gap exists only in states that chose not to expand Medicaid, leaving these individuals concentrated in southern states. They have essentially no options for health insurance. Another large group of the uninsured are the nearly 4 million undocumented immigrants, who are ineligible for coverage because of their documentation status.[51]

Overall, most uninsured Americans lack healthcare because they're poor. The United States does not guarantee health insurance, so those who can't afford it simply don't have it.

Even Americans with Health Insurance Can't Afford Healthcare—or They Pay Dearly for It

For too many Americans, seeing a doctor remains unaffordable even though they have health insurance. The raw number of people with health insurance does not tell the full story about how Americans are protected from healthcare costs: Americans are not just uninsured but *underinsured.* Researchers at the Commonwealth Fund track how many

Americans are underinsured, defined as carrying insurance with deductibles or out-of-pocket costs that rise above a certain threshold of income. Forty-five percent of nonelderly adults are either underinsured or uninsured—almost 90 million Americans.[52] In other words, nearly half of working-age Americans do not have adequate health insurance.

A third of Americans say that over the past year they or a family member have put off medical treatment due to cost. One in four Americans says they've put off treatment for a serious medical condition.[53] The proportion of Americans priced out of medical care for serious conditions has doubled since 2003. The percentage of people skipping doctor visits due to cost is three times higher in the United States than in our peer countries.

One reason Americans are being priced out of care is the trend toward higher deductibles in American health insurance, meaning that people need to pay more out of pocket before insurance kicks in. This trend hit Lisa and Dominic hard. Deductibles for covered workers doubled during the 2010s, and in 2019 the average annual deductible for a single person with job-based insurance was over $1,600.[54] Deductibles are even higher in the ACA marketplaces. In 2020, "silver" ACA plans had an average deductible of $4,300 for an individual and $8,820 for a family of four, and "bronze" ACA plans had an average deductible of $6,400 for an individual and $13,400 for a family of four.[55]

Unsurprisingly, these higher costs are a grave problem for Americans with low incomes and serious health needs.

Among low-income Americans with multiple chronic conditions enrolled in high-deductible plans, almost half spent more than 20 percent of total family income on out-of-pocket healthcare costs alone.[56] Women of all income levels on high-deductible plans experience months-long delays in getting breast cancer diagnosed and treated.[57]

Americans with insurance also suffer the costs of surprise medical bills. Patients often go to "in-network" hospitals but get treated by "out-of-network" physicians who haven't signed a deal with their insurance company. Other times, the ambulance that shows up when you call 911 isn't covered by your insurance. The result? Unexpected bills with potentially very high charges that insurance doesn't cover. More than two in five visits to the emergency room lead to a surprise bill. Beyond the emergency room, two in five hospital admissions come with an out-of-network charge, even when the hospital itself is in-network.[58] One in five patients who undergo an elective operation with an in-network surgeon also ends up with a surprise bill.[59] Lisa received her own surprise bill after the anesthesiologist who cared for her throughout one of her operations turned out to be outside her insurance network. In total, more than two in five Americans with health insurance say they or a family member has received an unexpected medical bill in the last two years.[60] Americans with health insurance simply can't be confident that their care will be covered.

All told, among sick Americans under age sixty-five—those who report being in fair or poor health—about half say they had trouble affording care in the last year.[61] Among Americans with serious illness, more than a third had healthcare costs so high that they spent *all or most of their savings* while sick.[62]

Patients on Medicare are not immune to these problems. The average Medicare enrollee spends over $3,000 a year out of their own pocket on medical bills.[63] For one in four seniors, medical costs consume more than 20 percent of total income. Medicare beneficiaries with serious illness fare even worse: more than half have had a serious problem paying their medical bills, more than a third used up most or all of their savings on medical expenses, and one in four were unable to pay for basic necessities.[64]

In today's America, health insurance doesn't make healthcare affordable, and it doesn't protect you from financial ruin.

Insurance Doesn't Cover All the Services Americans Need

Deductibles and out-of-pocket costs aren't the only reason that Americans with insurance can't access care. Oftentimes American health insurance simply doesn't cover certain services that are essential to health. Nearly 30 percent of Americans do not have dental insurance, including more than 60 percent of seniors.[65] Medicare today also does not cover vision, hearing, or long-term care services.

Furthermore, private insurers often maintain narrow provider networks as a cost containment tool; the result is that patients may not be able to seek care from the clinicians and hospitals best suited to their individual conditions. And even if patients receive care from an in-network provider, insurance companies often deny claims. For instance, in 2017 insurers on the ACA marketplaces denied one in five claims submitted.[66] Some insurance companies denied more than 40 percent of in-network claims.

Americans in Rural and Low-Income Urban Communities Have a Hard Time Getting Care

Health *insurance* is different from health *care*. Too many Americans in rural and low-income urban communities don't have access to care, even if they have insurance, because there simply aren't services in their communities.

One reason for this is hospital closures. Nearly 200 hospitals closed down between 2003 and 2011, and the shuttered hospitals were more likely to be safety-net hospitals that care for the poorest.[67] These closures have affected both urban and rural communities. And given the distances rural Americans have to travel to access services, a hospital shutdown can leave patients having to travel hours, even in emergency situations. It is significant that rural hospital closures have been concentrated in states that did not expand Medicaid, leaving more people uninsured and unable to pay for care. In these areas the harms of uninsurance spread to the entire community, which loses its ability to support a local health system.

Our fractured insurance system also creates special problems of access for patients on Medicaid. Doctors get paid less for seeing Medicaid patients: on average, Medicaid pays physicians 30 percent less than Medicare and about half as much as private insurance.[68] This means Medicaid patients have a harder time getting in to see a doctor. In one study, researchers posing as patients called thousands of doctors' offices and confirmed this disparity. If they said they had private insurance, they were turned away from an appointment just 14 percent of the time. But if they said they had Medicaid, they were turned away almost three times as often.[69]

There is also a national shortage of primary care doctors. Seventy-eight million Americans live in communities with primary care shortages.[70] This is largely because of the way we pay for primary care: the payment rates are low compared to specialty services, and in turn primary care doctors have significantly lower incomes than specialists. The income disparity is over $100,000 per year.[71] This means that when medical students look toward their future careers (and look toward paying off their medical school debt), they see that for a few years of extra training, they can increase lifetime earnings by several million dollars. They're responding to the incentives in the medical marketplace, and the result is too few primary care practitioners. The nationwide shortage of primary care doctors is particularly acute in low-income urban and rural areas, where more patients tend to be on Medicaid, which reimburses physicians at particularly low rates.[72]

American Healthcare Access Isn't Secure

Finally, American healthcare is precarious. Even Americans who have health insurance today can't be sure it will be there for them tomorrow. COVID-19 brought this insecurity into sharp relief, with early estimates indicating that over 5 million Americans lost their job-based coverage and became uninsured between February and May 2020 alone.[73] But American health insurance is insecure even in the best of times, with over 150 million Americans potentially just one pink slip away from losing healthcare for their entire family. In 2019, for instance—which was a strong year for the economy, by many measures—68 million Americans were separated from their jobs, including 21 million who were laid off.[74] Some people who lose their jobs qualify for Medicaid or subsidized insurance through the ACA. But millions do not, and those who do may find that coverage less than satisfactory: for instance, the high deductibles common in ACA plans are particularly hard to stomach after losing your income.

At best, tying health insurance to employment means Americans face red tape and administrative hoops when they move to a new workplace, and they may lose access to their doctors or medications. At worst, it means job loss can trigger a health crisis too, creating a toxic brew of economic and medical damage.

Even beyond health insurance, American healthcare institutions are themselves precarious. One of the most remarkable consequences of the COVID-19 pandemic was the way it choked off funding to our healthcare system during the worst public health crisis in a century. With fewer paying customers, nearly two thousand community health centers were forced to temporarily shut down.[75] Over a million healthcare workers lost their jobs between March and April 2020, including over 100,000 hospital workers.[76] As hospitals had to cancel their most lucrative elective services to prepare for the pandemic, some found themselves battling both COVID-19 and bankruptcy at the same time, sometimes losing the latter battle and shutting down at the peak of the pandemic when their communities relied on them most.[77]

For all these reasons, the most expensive healthcare system in the world is failing to provide adequate healthcare to all its people.

PROBLEM #3: AMERICANS ARE SICKER THAN WE SHOULD BE

Healthcare saves lives, so it should come as no surprise that access to it makes us healthier and lacking access makes us sicker. The clearest evidence on this point comes from studies showing that gaining health insurance prevents death. Numerous high-quality studies have found that Medicaid expansion has improved health and reduced mortality.[78] A recent study also provided the first evidence from a randomized trial—the gold standard of scientific evidence—that health insurance prevents death.[79] The Internal Revenue Service sent informational letters about health insurance options to millions of Americans who had previously paid a tax penalty for being uninsured under the ACA's individual mandate. Researchers found that Americans randomly chosen to receive the letter were more likely to have health insurance in subsequent years—and were less likely to die as a result. Estimates suggest that tens of thousands of Americans die every year due to lack of health insurance.[80]

Our Poor Health Is Driven by Severe Illness among the Poor and Marginalized

America as a whole has worse health outcomes than other wealthy countries. But these averages are driven by especially severe illness among the poor and marginalized: if you're poor or poorly educated, Black or Hispanic, the US healthcare system is stacked against you.

People with less than a high school education die seven years earlier than people with a university degree.[81] If you're poor in America, you also die earlier. And the gap between rich and poor is getting worse. Between 2001 and 2014, middle-income and high-income Americans gained an additional two years of life expectancy. But Americans in the bottom 5 percent of the income distribution had essentially no gains in survival.[82] The richest 1 percent of women live ten years longer than the poorest 1 percent of women, and the richest men live fifteen years longer than the poorest men.[83] Poverty affects not just how long you live but also your quality of life: compared to affluent adults, low-income adults with chronic illness are more than three times as likely to have limitations with routine activities like eating, bathing, and dressing.[84]

Black women die three years earlier than white women; Black men die almost five years earlier than white men.[85] Black and Hispanic women have higher rates of teenage pregnancy. Black mothers are more likely to give birth to preterm babies. Compared to babies of white mothers, babies of Black mothers are twice as likely to die before their first birthday. Black and Hispanic children have higher rates of obesity. Black men and women have the highest rates of hypertension. A large body of literature has shown us that this isn't because of anything essential about race, but because of structural, institutional, and interpersonal racism that has patterned education, income, and opportunity by race and ethnicity.

The Bigger Picture

The United States spends extraordinary sums of money on acute care after illness strikes. But our poor health is also driven by a relative lack of investment in the things that keep us well: primary care, preventive medicine, public health interventions, and social services.

It's true that Americans get some of the best care in the world when they're acutely ill—for instance, thirty-day survival rates after a heart attack or stroke are among the best in the world.[86] But given that Americans with these conditions still die earlier than their peers abroad, there's clearly something we're doing wrong before and after these catastrophic events. For instance, we have among the highest numbers of avoidable hospitalizations for diabetes and asthma, conditions where people can often avoid the hospital if their condition is well managed at home.

Furthermore, the root causes of illness frequently lie outside the healthcare system: too many Americans lack a safe home, healthy food, or social support. Unfortunately, we underinvest in social services like housing, public transit, and healthy-food subsidies that can help alleviate these social drivers of illness. International evidence suggests that increased social spending is associated with improvements in infant mortality, life expectancy, and premature mortality.[87] Although US healthcare spending is the highest in the world, our public sector spending on social services as a percentage of GDP is below average compared to other wealthy countries.[88] From this perspective, our lackluster health begins to look less surprising—particularly when you consider that much of the lag in our health outcomes is driven by illness among the poor, who rely most on publicly funded social services.

Any pathology in the wider society will imprint itself in people's bodies. Often policy in other domains negatively impacts health. Consider the obesity epidemic in America, which took off between the mid-1970s and early 1980s.[89] Since 1980, childhood obesity has tripled.[90] Did children's food and exercise preferences suddenly change in 1980? Did parents stop caring about their children's health? Probably not. In fact, recent polls have shown that obesity is one of the leading concerns that parents have about their kids' well-being, ranking at the top alongside bullying and drug use.[91]

Then what changed? The circumstances in which parents and children were making those choices. After food prices spiked in the early 1970s, the Nixon administration championed a policy of subsidizing corn in an attempt to bring prices down (and to help Nixon get reelected). The global price of corn dropped artificially. Suddenly corn became so ubiquitous that people found new uses for it: as a sweetener (high-fructose corn syrup), as a main source of feed for livestock, and even as a source of fuel for vehicles (ethanol blended with gasoline). American agricultural subsidies, particularly for corn and soy, have fundamentally changed the American foodscape—largely driving the growth of American food corporations like Coca-Cola, PepsiCo, Yum Foods, and McDonald's Corporation.

The American system of living also likely influences our health. Poor public transit coupled with suburban living and heavy reliance on automobiles decreases the amount of physical activity in daily life. And spread-out single-family homes can contribute to social isolation.

More broadly, nearly every challenge faced in American society—economic inequality, institutional racism, gun violence, loneliness, climate change, and more—impacts our health. Medical care and healthcare financing are critical, but it should come as no surprise that the project of improving human well-being is both deeper and broader.

Our System of Health Financing Hurts Poor and Marginalized People Worst

Reformers often separate health insurance and social determinants of health into two distinct categories: social factors are the upstream determinants of who gets sick in the first place, and health insurance allows you to get medical care if you get sick. But this view ignores the fact that our health financing system itself has a negative impact on the poorest and most marginalized people.

Take poverty, unemployment, food insecurity, and housing instability. These are all important social drivers of illness. Our health financing system contributes to all of them. Medical expenses push millions of Americans into poverty every year and contribute to hundreds of thousands of bankruptcies.[92] Poor health can make it difficult to find or keep work. High medical expenses eat into the family budget at large, making it harder to afford food and rent.

Improvements in healthcare financing have been shown to alleviate each of these drivers of illness. Medicaid expansion reduced poverty, bankruptcy filings, and medical debt; enrollees in Ohio and Michigan reported that it was easier to seek employment or continue working after they got insurance. Medicaid expansion also improved food security and reduced evictions.[93]

Adverse social determinants of health are powerful; the way we pay for healthcare makes them worse.

PROBLEM #4: THE EXPERIENCE OF GIVING AND RECEIVING HEALTHCARE IS ERODING

Virtually every American is (or will be) a patient of the healthcare system, and tens of millions of Americans are employed in healthcare. In our medical marketplace, patients and clinicians alike are getting left behind as our healthcare system becomes more complicated, more business-focused, and less personal.

Doctors Are Being Pushed Out of Independent Practice

As medical care becomes more sophisticated, it is increasingly necessary for primary care doctors, specialists, and hospitals to share information and communicate seamlessly. But American healthcare has taken this one step further, not just integrating information systems but actually allowing large hospitals to buy up other hospitals and practices to form giant consolidated conglomerates. Some proponents genuinely believe that the best healthcare system is the biggest healthcare system. But this consolidation is also driven by incentives in the private insurance system: bigger provider groups can leverage their market power to negotiate higher fees.

This corporate consolidation has made it harder and harder for independent healthcare practices to stay competitive, because when you get paid less for the same work compared to the giant health system across town, it's harder to hire staff and offer quality services. The number of physicians in solo practice has been steadily declining, while the number employed by hospitals or health systems is growing. Between 2012 and 2016, a whopping 36,000 physician practices were bought up by hospitals.[94] In 2018, only 31 percent of physicians identified themselves as independent practice owners or partners, down from nearly half in 2012.[95] This limits doctors' career options and erodes the autonomy that many physicians value highly.

Healthcare consolidation also means that physicians have relinquished more decision-making to health system administrators. Most doctors surveyed in 2018 said that physicians have little ability to significantly influence the healthcare system.[96] Meanwhile, doctors are spending nearly a quarter of their time on nonclinical paperwork, living out the administrative burden imposed by our complex and fragmented payment system.[97]

Consolidation Harms Nurses and Other Hospital Staff

Powerful hospital systems also put nurses and other staff at risk. The principle is the same as we've seen before: when there are few other options for employment, it's hard for staff to negotiate better wages or fair working conditions. For instance, hospital mergers have been found to decrease the wages of nursing and pharmacy workers.[98] Given this, it's no surprise that nurses' strikes are becoming so common. In September 2018, for example, over 7,000 nurses voted overwhelmingly to authorize a strike against Hospital Corporation of America, which owns more than 178 hospitals and is one of the largest hospital chains in the country.[99]

Moral Injury

Nurses, doctors, and other front-line clinicians confront the shortcomings of our healthcare system on a nearly daily basis. The consequence is *moral injury*: knowing what a patient needs but failing to meet that need because of barriers in the system. Large surveys have found that clinicians suffer high levels of moral distress when patients are unable to receive equitable care because they can't afford it—this includes nurses and physicians but extends to pharmacists, chaplains, and social workers as well.[100] Physician burnout is also a growing problem: nearly 80 percent of physicians say they experience burnout at least sometimes, and more than 40 percent say they experience burnout often or always.[101] Beyond contributing to burnout, moral injury marks the daily experience of tens of millions of Americans who have dedicated their careers to healthcare.

Patients Are Forced to Navigate a Maddeningly Complex Bureaucracy

Lisa's story shows the human toll exerted by our fragmented and expensive insurance system: there were times she felt more stressed by navigating the medical marketplace than she did by her husband's brain cancer diagnosis. Economist and Nobel laureate Richard Thaler refers to these exasperating bureaucratic hurdles as "sludge."[102] Patients spend untold hours wading through the sludge of our healthcare system just to get the care they need and deserve. Sometimes it is too much to overcome: one in four Americans reports missed or delayed care because of administrative burden.[103] Although researchers have focused on the burden that our bureaucratic healthcare system imposes on clinicians, the toll on patients and families is likely even larger.

This effect cannot be fully measured. Illness can have an immense impact on one's sense of identity and on the most important relationships in a person's life. Childbirth and the death of a loved one can be profound events. Americans are pulled away from these experiences to navigate the insurance bureaucracy, submit paperwork, fight coverage decisions, decipher medical bills, deplete their savings. Our healthcare system affects not just how we spend our money but how we spend our time at the most vulnerable and impactful junctures of our lives.

\\\\\\\\\\\\\\\\\\\\

That's the problem list we'll be focused on in this book. American healthcare is too expensive. Too many people can't get the care they need. We're sicker than we should be. And the experience of giving and receiving care is eroding.

Are these unrelated symptoms? Or are they common manifestations of the same underlying process?

There is a strong case to be made that America's unique healthcare problems stem from the unique structure of America's healthcare system, which is organized around a core principle: that healthcare should be treated as a consumer product.

Costs are high because healthcare does not have the fundamental characteristics of a market good, but we still buy and sell it in a marketplace—the resulting market failures keep prices high, and the marketplace itself imposes enormous administrative costs on the system. Poor and uneven access to care is an obvious consequence of treating healthcare as a consumer product: you receive as much care as you are willing and able to pay for, and the result is that millions go without needed care. We're sicker than our peers elsewhere in the world partly because our medical marketplace rations care according to income and fails to make investments that would keep us healthy over the long term. Our fragmented medical marketplace is also exhausting to navigate, eroding the experience of care for everyone involved.

To be sure, the American healthcare system contains some exceptions to the principle of treating healthcare as a consumer product. Every American is entitled to receive emergency care regardless of ability to pay—though they might receive an unaffordable bill in the mail after the fact. Seniors and some low-income Americans are guaranteed coverage from Medicare and Medicaid. But even these public programs have been injected with market features: most states have outsourced Medicaid to private insurance companies, and a third of Medicare beneficiaries are covered by private Medicare Advantage plans.

Most democracies have chosen to provide healthcare as a public good, available to all regardless of means. The United States generally provides healthcare as a market product, available to all who can afford it. But like the citizens of other democracies, many Americans over the last century have fought to make healthcare available to all. Why have we failed where others have succeeded?

2

HOW WE GOT HERE

A HISTORY OF HEALTH REFORM IN AMERICA

At present the United States has the unenviable distinction of being the only great industrial nation without compulsory health insurance.[1]

Economist Irving Fisher issued this indictment in 1916. More than a hundred years later, we remain the only wealthy nation without universal health coverage. How did we get here?

The American healthcare system is the product of a turbulent, century-long battle over who deserves healthcare, who pays, and who profits. That battle has been marked by conflict and compromise, good intentions and unfettered greed, calculated decisions and unintended consequences, idealism and defeat. In surprising ways, the story of health reform is woven into the story of America itself. But above all, it is an unfinished story.

In this chapter, we detail the series of attempts to pass healthcare reform legislation over the course of the twentieth and twenty-first centuries. These successes and failures shape the way the US healthcare system looks today and provide invaluable lessons on the barriers that future reform efforts will face—and how they might be overcome.

1912–1919: A PROGRESSIVE FAILURE

National health insurance first hit the American political conversation in 1912, when a group of reformers led by former president Theodore Roosevelt broke away from the Republican Party to form the Progressive Party. Nominating Roosevelt for the presidency, the Progressive Party included in its platform a call for "social insurance" to protect against the hazards of sickness.

European countries had already started to implement national health insurance. In 1883, Germany under Otto von Bismarck passed a "sickness insurance" scheme for German workers; Austria and Hungary followed suit soon after. In 1911, Great Britain passed the National Health Insurance Act, under which workers, employers, and the government paid into an insurance fund that would cover costs when a worker fell ill.

Today we think of health insurance as covering the costs of medical care, but the original purpose of "sickness insurance" was to protect against the risk of lost wages when an employee fell ill and couldn't work. This reflected economic reality: at the time, wage losses from illness were two to four times greater than medical costs.[2] Sickness was also the most common immediate cause of poverty.[3] If sickness threatened to destroy the livelihood of entire families, it seemed prudent to insure against it. The notion that healthcare itself would bankrupt Americans was still a long way off.

It seemed inevitable that the United States would follow its European counterparts in enacting health insurance. The *Journal of the American Medical Association* wrote that "experience in other countries has clearly demonstrated that in the course of a comparatively short time the question of social insurance will become an important issue in this country."[4]

Roosevelt lost the 1912 election, but reformers kept the movement for social insurance alive under the American Association for Labor Legislation (AALL), a progressive group composed largely of academics. In 1915 the AALL released a model health insurance bill, outlining a plan to cover medical expenses and lost wages. Similar to the German and British schemes, the cost of the insurance program would be split between workers, employers, and the government.

Foreshadowing the next century of health reform, the fate of the proposal was largely determined by the support and opposition of key interest groups: doctors, business, labor, and the insurance industry.

The American Medical Association (AMA) was initially sympathetic to the social insurance plan, reasoning that doctors and patients alike would benefit if more people could afford to pay for medical care. Praising European efforts to establish social insurance, the AMA's *Journal* wrote a glowing editorial in 1916: "No other social movement in modern economic development is so pregnant with benefit to the public."[5] This would be one of the last positive statements the AMA would make about expanding public health insurance for more than ninety years.

Doctors quickly turned against the AALL plan. Also foreshadowing the future, one of their chief concerns was their own pay. Physicians insisted that they should continue to be paid a separate fee for each service they provided, while reformers favored paying doctors a lump sum to cover all of a patient's care. Physicians also held the doctor-patient relationship in sacred regard and categorically opposed *any* third party getting involved in that relationship, including a third party whose job it was to pay the bills.

Businesses were opposed because they would be forced to pay into the workers' insurance fund, raising their costs. The budding insurance industry was also opposed. At that time, commercial insurance companies were focused on life insurance (including funeral benefits) rather than medical insurance. Because the AALL plan proposed to cover funeral benefits, insurance companies feared the plan would eat up a profitable line of business.

The labor movement had a complicated relationship with the AALL proposal. Whereas labor movements had been strong proponents of public health insurance in other countries, some American labor unions believed that the duty to provide insurance to workers lay with unions, not the government. Based on this reasoning, the American Federation of

Labor (AFL) was opposed to the insurance plan—although many within the AFL supported it.[6]

With a coalition of powerful stakeholders mobilized in opposition, the proposal for compulsory health insurance had dim prospects. World War I put a nail in the coffin. National priorities changed once America entered the war in 1917, and military warfare morphed into ideological warfare: opponents started to denounce national health insurance as a nefarious German plot.

Critically, the AALL plan also suffered from a lack of political leadership. The movement for compulsory health insurance was largely an outside effort, and it struggled to gain the legislative traction needed for passage.

Health reform failed in the 1910s, but Americans were still left with the problem of how to pay for medical care. Insurance companies were skeptical that health insurance could be a profitable business: the central problem was that people who choose to buy health insurance know they are likely to get sick, which means a lousy risk pool for the insurance company. The key innovation that allowed private health insurance to flourish was to scrap the idea of selling insurance to individuals and instead sell insurance to groups of employees. This not only provided a larger risk pool but also targeted workers who are likely to be younger and healthier than the population as a whole.

The turning point for private health insurance came in 1929. In exchange for an annual premium of $6 per person, Baylor University Hospital agreed to provide hospital care to a group of 1,500 schoolteachers in Dallas.[7] Eventually groups of hospitals in communities across the country banded together to offer these insurance products, and Blue Cross was born. Physicians were reluctant to take part in any insurance scheme, but eventually they decided voluntary insurance was acceptable so long as physicians were in charge of it, and Blue Shield emerged as insurance for physician services.

1932–1943: NO NEW DEAL FOR HEALTHCARE

When Franklin Delano Roosevelt (FDR) entered the White House after a landslide victory in 1932 during the worst economic depression to ever hit the United States, he quickly launched his ambitious New Deal. The legislative victories were impressive. Workers won the right to organize. The Works Progress Administration sent millions of Americans to work. Social Security provided seniors with a guaranteed pension.

What about healthcare? Nearly 70 percent of Americans thought it was a "good idea" for Social Security to pay for doctors' services and hospital care.[8] FDR instructed his advisors to prepare a proposal that would add healthcare to Social Security, but they had to keep it secret. Why? FDR feared that vitriolic opposition from the nation's doctors might tank the entire Social Security plan. "We can't go up against the State Medical Societies," FDR told a key Senate committee chairman. "We just can't do it."[9] Evidently, favorable public opinion was (and continues to be) not enough to secure the passage of health reform—or even to put it on the agenda.

The FDR era would nevertheless have a critical influence on the direction of American healthcare. An important factor is that during the New Deal the health insurance movement coalesced around a philosophy of reform: the goal was a universal, publicly funded program, available to all regardless of income. In essence, reformers wanted Social Security for healthcare. This public-good model of healthcare would dominate the health reform movement throughout the middle of the twentieth century.

But in a great irony, FDR also made a fateful decision that would solidify the central place of private, job-based health insurance in American life. During World War II, wartime production was rapidly driving up prices, and in response FDR instituted wage and price controls. But there was one catch: health benefits were exempted from the controls. Unable to raise wages, employers started offering health benefits as a way to attract workers. Even better, these health benefits were tax-free. (This tax break was confirmed by the Internal Revenue Code of 1954, signed by President Dwight Eisenhower.) In large measure, the dominance of employer-based insurance in the American healthcare system was the result of a historical accident.

1943–1950: DOCTORS EUTHANIZE NATIONAL HEALTH INSURANCE

After FDR's passing, national health insurance would find a political champion in his vice president and successor in the White House, Harry Truman. National health insurance was

Truman's first domestic policy priority, making him the first sitting president in American history to give a full-throated endorsement of single-payer national health insurance.

Truman's plans were buoyed by a movement for national health insurance that already existed within the US Congress. Beginning in 1943, a trio of legislators sponsored a series of bills—the Wagner-Murray-Dingell bills—that served as the first serious legislative proposals for single-payer healthcare in US history.

Learning from past failures, both Truman and congressional leaders understood the importance of winning the support of doctors. They were also aware of how doctors had smeared public insurance as "socialized medicine" throughout the 1930s, framing the issue as a question of "Americanism versus Sovietism."[10]

To appease the medical profession, Truman said he would "pay doctors more than the best they have received in peacetime years." After the national health insurance bill was introduced, Senator Robert Wagner wrote a letter to the AMA's *Journal* explaining: "There is absolutely no intention on the part of the authors to 'socialize' medicine, nor does the bill do so. We are opposed to socialized medicine or to state medicine. The health insurance provisions of the bill are intended simply to provide a method of paying medical costs in advance and in small convenient amounts."[11]

But the AMA was vitriolic in its opposition. They suggested that national health insurance would make the surgeon general of the United States more powerful than a Nazi leader, and that it would make doctors "slaves."[12]

Congressional opponents sounded similar alarms. Republican senator Robert Taft suggested that compulsory health insurance came right out of the Soviet constitution.[13] A House subcommittee insinuated that proponents of national health insurance included "known Communists" pursuing "the Moscow party line."[14]

Though he was the incumbent, Truman's election prospects were dim in the 1948 presidential race, and Republican control of Congress meant that national health insurance was all but dead. In an attempt to turn the tide, Truman doubled down on national health insurance during his campaign. In one of the great upsets in American electoral history, Truman defeated Republican Thomas Dewey. It was a blue wave: Democrats retook both chambers of Congress (including gaining more than seventy-five seats in the House), and rising star Lyndon B. Johnson won a seat in the Senate. With a united Democratic government and a president who placed national health insurance at the center of his campaign, the prospects of single-payer healthcare—snatched from the jaws of defeat—looked unexpectedly bright.

But doctors panicked. The AMA hired Campaigns, Inc., a public relations firm that rose to prominence after successfully destroying a universal healthcare proposal in California. The AMA levied an annual $25 fee on its members to fund its opposition efforts, and ultimately raised a $3.5 million war chest (nearly $40 million in today's dollars) to fund its smear campaign.[15] It was the most expensive lobbying campaign the nation had ever seen.[16]

It was an all-out assault. The AMA and Campaigns, Inc. worked to get everything and everyone aligned against Truman's plan—they deployed public speakers, pamphlets, the press, private organizations, and more. One pamphlet read: "Would socialized medicine lead to the socialization of other phases of American life? Lenin thought so. He declared: 'Socialized medicine is the keystone to the arch of the Socialist State.'"[17] (The Lenin quote was apparently fabricated; the Library of Congress was unable to find it in Lenin's speeches.)

The AMA's campaign to destroy national health insurance was supported by a coalition of wealthy interests including insurance companies, pharmaceutical companies, and big business. The Committee for the Nation's Health, a group in support of the reform effort, spent $36,000 in 1950—compared to over $2 million spent in opposition by the AMA, including an outlay of $1 million in the two weeks before the congressional elections, when "every bona fide weekly and daily newspaper in the United States (10,033 in all) carried a five-column-wide, fourteen-inch-deep ad from the AMA or from one of its business allies decrying the enemies of free enterprise, while 1600 radio stations broadcast spot announcements and 35 magazines carried similar advertisements."[18]

Public support withered from 58 percent to 36 percent.[19] Three-quarters of Americans who knew about Truman's health plan were aware of the AMA's opposition. The reform failed, and the movement for public health insurance would stay quiet over the next decade.

The AMA and its allies were the most conspicuous opponents of national health insurance, but Truman's effort faced an equally important barrier: conservative Democrats in Congress. The Democratic Party of the day was home not just for liberals but also for conservatives from the segregated South. Although Democrats held large majorities in Congress after the 1948 election, in practice the conservative coalition of Republicans and southern Democrats posed a formidable obstacle to the passage of Truman's policy agenda.[20] These twin barriers—well-funded interest group opposition and conservative congressional Democrats—would need to be overcome to pass any major expansion of health insurance.

1959–1965: MEDICARE FOR SOME

Stung by the defeat of Truman's national health plan, reformers quickly formulated a new strategy: focus only on hospital insurance for seniors. "We all saw insurance for the elderly as a fallback position, which we advocated solely because it seemed to have the best chance politically," writes Robert Ball, a top official in the Kennedy and Johnson administrations. "We expected Medicare to be a first step toward universal national health insurance."[21]

This compromise plan maintained the New Deal reform philosophy—health insurance should be provided as a social good, available regardless of income—but narrowed its scope in order to maximize its political acceptability. Seniors were viewed sympathetically as a group suffering greatly from lack of insurance and focusing only on hospital services (rather than physician care) might avoid the ire of the AMA. Reformers were still committed to national health insurance as a long-term goal, but hospital insurance for seniors looked to be the best place to start.[22]

There was also an economic logic to this focus. Hospital prices had doubled during the 1950s, but the job-based private insurance industry left seniors with little ability to secure affordable health coverage.[23] More than half of retirees had no form of health insurance.[24] Since seniors were a group that private insurers were less eager to cover—age is one of the best predictors of medical problems, making older people less profitable for insurers—targeting a government program at seniors might also arouse less opposition from the insurance industry.

John F. Kennedy made hospital insurance for seniors—which started to be called Medicare—a key part of his successful 1960 presidential campaign. In 1961, all the pieces seemed to be in place for successful health reform. A popular president had just been elected. Democrats had large majorities in both chambers of Congress. There was broad consensus on a specific approach to reform. And an overwhelming two-thirds majority of the public supported Medicare.[25]

But JFK confronted the same obstacle as Truman: conservative Democrats in Congress. In particular, southern Democrats who opposed Medicare had control of the congressional committee responsible for the bill. Congressman Wilbur Mills, a fiscally conservative Democrat from Arkansas, was chair of the powerful Ways and Means Committee and had already blocked Medicare bills in 1959 and 1960.[26] In the midst of the civil rights movement, Medicare also suffered opposition from segregationist Democrats who worried that a federal health insurance program would lead to the government forcing southern hospitals to integrate.

A further difficulty was hostility from physicians, who continued their legacy as the perennial opponents of health reform. In 1961, the AMA commissioned the actor Ronald Reagan to record a screed against Medicare, in which he denounced the hospital insurance program as "socialized medicine." Reagan warned that if Medicare passes, "we are going to spend our sunset years telling our children, and our children's children, what it once was like in America when men were free."

The AMA was also willing to use more clandestine tactics to undermine Medicare. By 1964, it looked like the Medicare bill might have a chance. Congressman John Watts, a southern Democrat, had decided to support Medicare, which would give the bill the key vote it needed to make it out of committee. But the day before the vote, he reversed his position in what looks like a stunning backroom conspiracy.

Earlier that year, the first surgeon general's report on smoking was released, and its conclusions were unambiguous: heavy smokers were twenty times more likely than nonsmokers to develop lung cancer. Tobacco companies panicked—and the AMA seemingly saw an opportunity for a deal. The historical record can't prove a quid pro quo, but the facts are alarming. The AMA argued that the surgeon general's report was "inconclusive," and it released its own information claiming that some equally competent physicians advise to "smoke if you feel you should, but be moderate." Meanwhile, Congressman Watts from Kentucky, a tobacco-growing state, reversed his Medicare vote. Another congressman from New Jersey connected the dots: "The AMA has made a deal with the tobacco industry . . . to get tobacco-state congressmen to vote against Medicare. It's an outrage."[27]

The failure of Medicare during JFK's presidency highlights a foundational challenge for health reform: American political institutions are highly resistant to change. Contrast our system of checks and balances with the parliamentary democracies of western Europe. In a parliamentary system, massive electoral victories can lead to swift enactment of a political party's major policy initiatives—especially if a specific policy has broad public support. The American political system has more barriers to change, with a president elected separately from the legislature, two distinct chambers of Congress elected in different ways (and on different timelines), and various procedural and committee rules that diffuse power across different elected actors. Each of these roadblocks also give powerful interest groups an opportunity to block reform. Opponents to health reform can stop a law by blocking it at a single juncture; proponents often must string together compromise after compromise, success after success to shepherd reform through a treacherous political maze.

How did Medicare eventually overcome congressional deadlock and opposition from powerful interest groups? One important factor is that Medicare was the first health insurance movement that enjoyed significant grassroots support.[28] A Senate subcommittee on aging held hearings across the country in 1959, and "the old folks lined up by the dozen everyplace we went."[29] Their primary concern was overwhelmingly clear: medical care. One magazine reported that the pressure to take action was "assuming the proportions of a crusade."[30] The labor movement was also a powerful organizing force for Medicare, with the AFL-CIO providing a counterweight to the AMA in public debate.[31]

The turning point came at the ballot box. Public support for Medicare remained consistently high through the early 1960s, and effective organizing by seniors and the labor movement was able to translate this support into electoral victories.[32] The 1964 election was a landslide. Lyndon B. Johnson (LBJ) upended conservative Barry Goldwater, winning by the largest margin in a presidential election since 1820. Democrats gained the largest majorities in the House and Senate since the New Deal. Crucially, the new Democratic majority brought in enough liberals to overwhelm the conservative coalition of Republicans and southern Democrats that had stymied reform for decades. LBJ, who had served in Congress for over twenty years and earned a reputation as the "master of the Senate," was ready to deploy his legendary legislative acumen to push for Medicare.

Wilbur Mills, the congressman who had blocked Medicare so many times before, saw the writing on the wall. So did the AMA. And as would happen many times in the future, when comprehensive reform seemed inevitable, interest groups offered a watered-down alternative. In this case, the AMA proposed expanding a state-run program for the elderly poor, rather than enacting a universal program for seniors. Republicans offered another alternative: physician insurance for seniors, offered by the government on a voluntary basis.

With reform seemingly inevitable, Wilbur Mills made a stunning move: instead of choosing among the three plans, he *combined* them. The Mills bill was a "three-layered cake": the original Democratic proposal for Medicare became Medicare Part A, covering hospital care as part of Social Security; the Republican proposal became Medicare Part B, covering physician services; the AMA proposal became Medicaid, a state-run program for the poor. Wilbur Cohen, a leader in the Kennedy and Johnson administrations who was instrumental in developing Medicare, lauded Mills's three-layered cake as "the most brilliant legislative move I'd seen in 30 years . . . Mills had taken the AMA's ammunition, put it in the Republicans' gun, and blown them both off the map."[33]

When Mills brought the unified bill to the floor of the House in 1965, he received a standing ovation. The chief opponent to Medicare had become its lasting champion—though only after a historic election forced his hand.

Lyndon Johnson traveled to an unexpected place to sign the historic bill into law a few months later: Independence, Missouri. He chose that location so he could invite a special guest to join him at the table for the signing: eighty-one-year-old Harry Truman, the first president to champion national health insurance. America still did not have universal health insurance, but at the stroke of a pen, nearly every American older than sixty-five was covered. Medicare would also eventually compel southern hospitals to integrate, a major win in the fight for civil rights.

The bill creating Medicare and Medicaid was the single most important piece of healthcare legislation in American history—nothing before or since has come close to the scale of its achievement. But its legacy is complicated. Politically, by segmenting off specific groups for health coverage, Medicare and Medicaid undermined a more unified movement for national health insurance—those with government insurance became key opponents to expansion, fearing it might compromise their own coverage. Indeed, sociologist Paul Starr identifies this "protected public" as an important source of opposition to comprehensive health reform.[34]

Furthermore, healthcare costs exploded after Medicare was implemented. Of course, some increase in spending was intended: seniors were able to use services they previously had not had access to. But the cost explosion was also the result of major policy failure. Eschewing any efforts at cost control, legislators essentially allowed providers to charge the government whatever prices they wanted. It was the "blank check" method of health policy. Controlling this cost explosion would set the stage for future reform battles, diverting attention away from further expansions in coverage.

1971–1974: TED KENNEDY VS. RICHARD NIXON

President Richard Nixon was deeply concerned about the rising cost of healthcare. "We face a massive crisis in this area," he warned. "Unless action is taken . . . within the next two to three years, we will have a breakdown in our medical care system."[35] Hospital costs were increasing at 14 percent a year.[36] The "reasonable and customary" fees providers agreed to charge were ballooning. Everyone footing the bill for expensive healthcare started to band together: government, business, and insurance companies formed a coalition against providers. It was a rare opportunity to enact major reform. Which path would reformers take?

Senator Ted Kennedy was the most prominent advocate for universal health insurance in the second half of the twentieth century. In the 1970s, he led the second major movement in American history for single-payer healthcare. He championed the Health Security Act in 1971, which would have enacted a universal national health insurance system.

President Richard Nixon feared that Ted Kennedy would challenge him for the presidency in 1972 with healthcare as his key campaign issue. Nixon decided to meet this challenge head-on, proposing the most comprehensive federal health reform plan of any modern Republican president. By 1974, Nixon said that comprehensive health insurance was an "idea whose time has come in America." His plan was sweeping: he proposed universal coverage through a combination of government-subsidized insurance, private employer coverage, and Medicare.

Kennedy's national health insurance plan faced off against Nixon's public-private mix. Neither would win.

Aides for Nixon and Kennedy held a secret meeting in a church basement in Washington, DC, to hammer out a compromise, but neither side would accept it. The Nixon administration insisted that Kennedy accept private insurance companies as the central source of coverage for most working adults. Kennedy, who had already started to alienate his base by compromising on his original single-payer plan, couldn't do it. After the failed attempt at compromise, a *New York Times* headline summed up the situation: "A Legislative Goal That Has No Foes Stalled by Differences in Approach."[37]

In retrospect, Nixon's public-private plan was remarkably similar to the Affordable Care Act (ACA) passed under President Obama. Both the Nixon plan and the ACA keep Medicare in place and require employers to offer health insurance to their employees.[38] For everyone else, the ACA expanded coverage through a combination of Medicaid expansion and subsidized private insurance; similarly, under the Nixon plan every citizen not on Medicare or employer coverage would be offered an insurance plan subsidized by the government.[39]

In the 1970s, this public-private approach to health reform was a Republican plan, with Democrats unwilling to stomach the compromise. By the 2000s, the public-private approach was a Democratic plan, garnering not a single Republican vote.

The demise of national health insurance in the 1970s coincided with a national political transformation. In 1980, Ronald Reagan won the presidency in a decisive victory, ushering in a new era in American politics. The imagery is powerful: Reagan, the actor who fiercely and famously opposed Medicare in the 1960s, was chosen by an overwhelming majority of Americans to run the federal government. The New Deal liberalism that had dominated the twentieth century was replaced by Reagan's vision for small government, individual liberty, and market solutions.

The health reform movement was swept up in this shift. For most of the century, health reformers were driven by a commitment to social insurance—coverage ought to be provided by government as a universal public good. From the Reagan era through the Obama presidency, the dominant philosophy was that government should create the right conditions for private companies to provide health insurance as a market good.

1980S: HEALTHCARE, INC.

The healthcare debate in the 1980s was dominated not by how to expand coverage but by how to control costs. Medical advances contributed to an explosion in healthcare costs throughout the middle of the century, and there was no countervailing force to keep spending in check: Medicare gave providers free rein to charge whatever prices they pleased, and insurance companies were too fractured to restrain price increases in the private market.

Perhaps ironically, Reagan—the ultimate champion of the free market—initiated the first effective measure of federal government price regulation in healthcare. In 1983, Medicare ended its "blank check" method of reimbursing hospitals, where Medicare would cover whatever costs the hospital reported. Instead, Medicare would pay hospitals a predetermined sum every time they admitted a Medicare patient, with the amount depending on the patient's diagnosis—this gave hospitals an incentive to constrain costs per admission, rather than spend lavishly on the taxpayer's dime.[40] In 1989, Medicare also began to regulate how it paid physicians, setting up a fee schedule for various services rather than accepting whatever rates the physician billed.

Increasingly effective regulation in Medicare occurred alongside deregulation of private healthcare markets. In

1980, thirty states had some sort of rate regulation or budget review for hospitals.[41] Throughout the 1980s and early 1990s, nearly every state abandoned these efforts, leaving an unfettered market for the prices that hospitals could charge to private insurers.

For hospitals, this environment created a clear business strategy: get bigger. With stable Medicare rates and a newly deregulated private market, the most effective way to increase revenue was to command higher prices from privately insured patients. The best way to do this was to build monopoly power. Especially with a lax antitrust environment (federal antitrust enforcers lost six cases in a row attempting to challenge healthcare mergers in the 1990s), a wave of hospital consolidation took off.[42]

This era also brought a shift in the way the country thought and talked about healthcare. As Rashi Fein, an economist who helped design Medicare, wrote in 1982: "A new language is infecting the culture of American medicine. It is the language of the marketplace, of the tradesman, and of the cost accountant. It is a language that depersonalizes both patients and physicians and describes medical care as just another commodity."[43]

Physicians and patients became providers and consumers. Some reformers lauded this market-based turn as the missing ingredient needed to control American healthcare costs. But Fein was troubled: "A decent medical-care system that helps all the people cannot be built without the language of equity and care. If this language is permitted to die and is completely replaced by the language of efficiency and cost control, all of us—including physicians—will lose something precious."

1993: THE CLINTONS' DISASTER

Health insurance returned to the national spotlight as a top priority for President Bill Clinton. After nearly two decades on the back burner, in the early 1990s health reform had an aura of inevitability. Skyrocketing healthcare costs once again paved the way for an alignment of business and government interests, as ballooning costs increasingly ate into corporate balance sheets and government budgets alike. Yet again, the question seemed to be not whether health reform would happen but what form it would take.

The form of Clinton's health proposal was shaped by his political ideology. A product of the rightward shift in American politics, Clinton was a "New Democrat" who sought to combine conservative-leaning fiscal policy with liberal-leaning social policy, searching for a "Third Way" to navigate the traditional divide between liberals and conservatives.

As such, Clinton's healthcare plan was a complex attempt to appeal to liberals through universal coverage and to conservatives through private market competition. Known as "managed competition within a budget," the Clinton plan would have provided guaranteed access to a private insurance plan, which was chosen from a highly regulated marketplace run by each state and funded by contributions from employers.

Three forces conspired to kill the Clinton plan: the loss of stakeholder support, startlingly effective insurance industry attack ads, and scorched-earth Republican opposition.

To begin with, support for the Clinton plan was mixed among important interest groups. Doctors and hospitals initially supported the concept of health reform, but they were turned off when cost control measures were introduced.[44] Businesses offered mixed support at the start, but they eventually turned against the plan. Large insurance companies actually supported the plan, because it would effectively call on large insurers to provide universal coverage, greatly expanding their customer base. But smaller insurance companies saw the plan as an existential threat, thinking they would be forced to fold under a proposed market structure that favored large plans. So they went on the attack.

Enter Harry and Louise, the unassuming middle-aged stars of a television ad campaign against the Clinton plan. Americans across the country watched their conversation across a kitchen table:

ANNOUNCER: *Times are changing, and not all for the better. The government may force us to pick from a few healthcare plans designed by government bureaucrats.*

LOUISE: *Having choices we don't like is no choice at all.*

HARRY: *If they choose . . .*

LOUISE: *We lose.*

The trade group representing these insurance companies spent over $15 million to bring Harry and Louise to American televisions. (It was a good investment: the ads brought in an additional $20 million in contributions.) In total, the insurance companies spent over $50 million to defeat Clinton's health plan—an even greater fortune than the AMA had spent razing the Truman effort half a century prior. The ad campaign was a national sensation, and Harry and Louise became household names. Senator Jay Rockefeller called it "the single most destructive campaign I've seen in over thirty years."[45]

The other development that helped defeat the Clinton plan was a new strategy of all-out opposition by congressional Republicans, led by Newt Gingrich. As explained by health policy experts Stuart Altman and David Shactman, "For the first time in many years . . . it became acceptable, in matters of national significance, to oppose legislation not on its merits, but simply to deny an accomplishment of the opposing political party."[46] Given political polarization in the modern era, this style of politics may seem so commonplace that it's difficult to imagine any other way of governing. But Clinton's healthcare plan was premised on the idea that he would be able to win over moderate Republican votes, even if he lost some Democrats. But as would happen with the Affordable Care Act, the idea that health coverage could be expanded with bipartisan support proved to be nothing more than naive fantasy.

As conservative strategist Bill Kristol put it, the plan's success would "help Democratic prospects in 1996. But the long-term political effects of a successful Clinton health care bill will be even worse—much worse . . . it will revive the reputation of the [Democratic Party] as the generous protector of middle-class interests."[47] In short, one Republican argument against national health reform wasn't that it would hurt the American people. Even scarier: it might help them, and Democrats would get the credit.

Finally, Democrats were hampered because they were in internal disarray. President Clinton made health reform a centralized (and secretive) effort run from the White House—spearheaded by First Lady Hillary Rodham Clinton—rather than letting Congress take the lead. (As a former governor, President Clinton seemed to lack the legislative instincts deployed so masterfully by Lyndon Johnson.) Meanwhile, Congress debated several bills simultaneously with no agreement on which path to take. Clinton's eventual plan was based on a complex proposal crafted by academic economists and refined by a massive team of elite policy analysts. Policy merits aside, the Clinton plan was difficult to message or explain to the American people.

Furthermore, the Clinton plan had political leadership but was divorced from any national movement pushing for that approach to reform. There was consensus that reform was needed, but "managed competition within a budget" risked being seen as a technocratic non sequitur, lacking clarity on which problems were being tackled and how. Contrast that with Medicare, where an organized national movement coalesced around the specific idea of publicly financed hospital insurance for seniors.

Despite the aura of inevitability, the Clinton plan died without reaching a vote. Its failure provides a classic case study in how health reform fails in America.[48] Glaring deficiencies in our healthcare system create widespread demands for change. Politicians make health reform a priority and win elections. Public opinion starts out high. Then health reform enters the legislative process, inevitably hitting snags and delays as the details are debated and alternative approaches are offered. Opponents raise money from all the industry groups who have a financial interest in maintaining the status quo. They build a united front and exploit disagreements among factions of reformers. They use their war chest to fund advertising campaigns intended to stoke fears of change and paint reform as an expensive government overreach. Public support dwindles. Politicians get cold feet and abandon the effort.

Next time around, reformers were determined to avoid this well-worn path to failure. Their central strategy: prevent the healthcare industry from tanking reform by proposing a plan that the industry supports.

2008–2010: AN EPIC BATTLE FOR INCREMENTAL REFORM

The design of the Affordable Care Act began even before Barack Obama won the presidency in 2008. Behind the scenes, groups of strange bedfellows were already working together to craft the broad outlines for the next Democratic healthcare reform effort. Smarting from a string of losses—especially the failure of the Clinton plan—the early consensus was to take the middle road, attempting to expand coverage while disturbing key stakeholders as little as possible.

The ACA was a complex piece of legislation, but its two strategies to expand health insurance were relatively straightforward. The first was expanding the Medicaid program to cover *everyone* under a certain percentage of the federal poverty line (rather than limiting the program to specific groups of the poor, like pregnant mothers or people with disabilities). For those above that income level, the second strategy was creating marketplaces for individuals to buy private health insurance. Just like consumers can go to websites like Google Flights or Expedia to shop for airline tickets sold by private companies, the idea was that consumers could go to HealthCare.gov (or the state equivalent) to shop for health plans sold by private companies.

Traditionally, most individuals who chose to purchase individual health insurance were quite sick, so premiums were very high. To guard against this, insurers adopted the hated practice of denying coverage to people with preexisting conditions. This created the awful problem where people who needed insurance the most—those with conditions like cancer, heart disease, or depression—were being denied the opportunity to buy it.

To solve this problem, the ACA marketplaces were supported by a "three-legged stool."[49] First, insurance companies were no longer allowed to deny coverage to people with preexisting conditions. Second was a mandate for individuals to buy health insurance or face a financial penalty. The mandate was intended to bring healthy people into the risk pool and keep premiums under control as people with preexisting conditions entered the market. Third were subsidies to help low-income people buy insurance on the marketplaces, because otherwise the mandated purchase of health insurance would be financially difficult for them.

In designing, refining, and proposing these policies, the Obama reform effort is notable for its early and active effort to engage key healthcare stakeholders. Obama sought to strike deals with drug companies, insurance companies, hospitals, and the AMA.

In a secret deal, the administration secured the support of the Pharmaceutical Research and Manufacturers of America (PhRMA)—the pharmaceutical lobby—by promising to block any provision that would allow Medicare to negotiate drug prices.[50] In exchange, PhRMA promised to give certain voluntary discounts on prescription drugs. PhRMA announced their support of the Obama plan early on.

Since hospitals would benefit from newly insured patients, the administration wanted hospitals to help cover part of the cost of expanding coverage. The administration made a deal with the hospital industry that hospitals would accept a $200 billion reduction in payments from government programs over ten years (largely from Medicare), on the theory that hospitals would bring in new revenue from the millions of Americans who would gain insurance. But this deal did not affect all hospitals equally: hospitals that treated fewer uninsured patients would lose more than they gained under the proposal. Furthermore, hospitals were opposed to the "public option"—a government healthcare plan to be sold alongside the private plans—because they feared the public plan would enable the government to set payment rates lower than they could negotiate with private insurers. In the end, the hospitals would come around to support reform—but only after the public option was removed, and after hospitals were exempted from a key cost control measure that had been included in the original plan.[51]

It looked like the insurance companies might be on board with reform, too. One might think that a government requirement for all Americans to buy your product would be an attractive deal. But insurance companies objected vehemently to the public option, and also opposed the "80/20 rule," which required insurance companies to spend at least 80 percent of revenues on medical claims (as opposed to administration and profit). But even after the public option was dropped, insurers opposed the final legislation and helped funnel money into television ads attacking the plan.[52]

That left the perennial opponents of health reform: doctors. Democratic leadership attempted to woo doctors by offering to boost their pay. Senator Harry

Reid promised the AMA that he would introduce separate legislation to repeal scheduled payment reductions to doctors, even though the measure would cost the government over $200 billion. He also promised to increase the doctors' fee schedule by half a percentage point. In return, the doctors were told that the administration "needed and expected their support."[53] Though the AMA wanted other concessions, once they saw that reform was inevitable, they chipped in their support.

It turned out to be a stable coalition: doctors, hospitals, and drug companies in support, insurance companies opposed.

But healthcare interests weren't the only flash points in the ACA debate. The Obamacare debates also demonstrated how health reform can become entangled in partisan warfare during times of tremendous political polarization.

Despite the ACA's deliberately incremental nature, opponents hurled ideological attacks against it, calling it a "government takeover of healthcare." Media coverage fixated on nonexistent "death panels," a claim made by former vice presidential candidate Sarah Palin that the ACA would force Americans to stand before a panel of government bureaucrats who would decide if they are worthy of healthcare. Illegal immigration was briefly used as an attack against the ACA, even though the plan did very little to help undocumented immigrants. Finally, controversy about funding for abortion almost killed the plan on more than one occasion, with pro-life Democrats nearly willing to let the whole plan sink rather than vote for a bill that made it look like taxpayer money was being used to cover abortion services.

The failure of bipartisanship is also deeply instructive. From the beginning, the ACA was designed to be a bipartisan compromise. The individual mandate had its roots in a 1989 paper from the conservative Heritage Foundation which framed the requirement as a matter of personal responsibility.[54] In 2008, a health insurance bill that featured the individual mandate was supported by nine Republican and nine Democratic senators. [55] The ACA was also explicitly modeled on "Romneycare," the Massachusetts reform plan championed by Republican governor Mitt Romney. The ideological character of the ACA also seemed to square with conservative principles, as it relied on a competitive marketplace of private insurance plans. If Republicans were going to support a near-universal healthcare proposal, this seemed to be it.

But the forces of polarization were simply too strong. Once the ACA became a signature effort of Obama and the Democrats—with Romneycare now rebranded as Obamacare—Republicans became vitriolic opponents to the law. Echoing the strategy of all-out opposition deployed against the Clinton reform, a Republican senator explained, "If we're able to stop Obama on this it will be his Waterloo. It will break him."[56]

The ACA passed without a single Republican vote. The Democratic Party—the party of FDR, Harry Truman,

Lyndon Johnson, and Ted Kennedy—found themselves defending market-based health reform against Republican attacks. The Republican Party, having decided that the ACA approach was anathema, left themselves with limited space in the future to craft a distinctive vision for expanding health coverage.

In the end, the greatest political strength of the ACA was its tremendous effort to win the support of major healthcare stakeholders. But that was also its biggest policy weakness. Ironically, one of the ACA's most fundamental policy decisions was to accommodate the private insurance industry: leave the current employer-based system entirely in place and add a requirement for more people to buy private insurance. But the insurance industry *still* opposed the ACA. Furthermore, the ACA was unable to pursue many effective cost-control strategies because of the compromises made to win political support: avoiding any significant efforts to control drug prices, exempting hospitals from cost control measures, ramping up payments to doctors, and leaving out a public option.

When the ACA was passed in 2010, nearly 47 million Americans were uninsured. The ACA helped more than 40 percent of those people get covered, and by 2016 the number of Americans without insurance reached a new low of 27 million.[57] Despite its incremental nature, the Affordable Care Act is undoubtedly the most successful effort to expand healthcare coverage since Medicare.

2011–2020: HEALTH INSECURITY AND THE RISE OF MEDICARE FOR ALL

Despite the coverage gains made by the Affordable Care Act, the 2010s were a decade that brought growing health insecurity for a broad swath of Americans.

Continued political battles around the ACA provided one source of insecurity. The Supreme Court ruled that Medicaid expansion must be optional for states, not universal. Many red-state governments either declined to expand Medicaid or sought new ways to restrict enrollment. The 2016 election brought in a president and a new crop of legislators promising to repeal and replace the ACA; that effort ultimately failed, but the ACA's mandate for individuals to purchase health insurance was functionally repealed. At the dawn of 2020, the ACA was mired in yet another legal battle.

While political attention was focused on Medicaid and the ACA marketplaces, the job-based insurance market continued to erode. Prices jumped. Premiums rose. Deductibles soared.

Middle-class Americans with stable jobs learned they were no longer protected from financial disaster if illness struck. Through social media, Americans who remained healthy gained an uncomfortable front-row seat to the suffering of their neighbors. Even among Americans with insurance, journalists uncovered heartbreaking stories of young people with diabetes rationing insulin, families with sick children having their wages seized, mothers with cancer imprisoned after missing court dates for unpaid medical bills.[58] The next round of health reform would need to include relief for Americans *with* health insurance, too.

With a growing appetite for new solutions, Medicare for All rapidly became a centerpiece of the health reform debate. Bernie Sanders's outsider campaign for the presidency in 2016 catalyzed the resurgence of national health insurance in the American political conversation. After successfully beating back ACA repeal efforts in 2017, Democrats needed a positive vision for how to move forward on health reform; the burgeoning progressive movement lifted up Medicare for All as a leading option to claim that mantle.

After decades on the fringes of political discourse, Medicare for All was embraced by elected officials at astonishing speed. When Congressman John Conyers introduced the first Medicare for All bill in the House of Representatives in 2003, it had thirty-eight cosponsors; by the 2017–18 Congress, it had 124. Similarly, when Senator Ted Kennedy first introduced a Medicare for All bill in the Senate in 2006, it gained zero cosponsors. When Senator Sanders introduced a version in 2017, 16 senators signed on. In the 2018 midterm elections, nearly 50 percent of Democrats contesting seats in the House of Representatives endorsed Medicare for All.[59] In 2019, Congress held four hearings on Medicare for All, including in the powerful Ways and Means Committee—the same lawmaking body that had blocked Medicare legislation sixty years earlier before championing it.

Medicare for All also became a key flash point in the 2020 Democratic primary campaign. Senators Bernie Sanders and Elizabeth Warren were the leading proponents of the policy. Other front-runners stopped short of endorsing Medicare for All, but a consensus began to emerge in the Democratic Party that the appropriate way to expand health coverage was to extend some version of Medicare to more people—a remarkable transformation for a party whose signature policy achievement a decade earlier had hinged on subsidizing a new marketplace of private insurance plans. Democratic primary voters ultimately nominated as their candidate for the presidency Joe Biden, who did not support Medicare for All. Still, Democratic voters favored Medicare for All by a wide margin: in twenty-two out of twenty-three states where CNN conducted polls of Democratic primary voters, the majority said they preferred "a government plan for all instead of private insurance." (The only exception was South Carolina, where 49 percent were in support versus 46 percent opposed.) In some states, including Illinois and Maine, exit polls suggested that most Democrats who voted for Joe Biden in the primary also supported Medicare for All.[60]

To gauge public support nationally, the Kaiser Family Foundation conducted fifteen polls from 2017 through May 2020 on Medicare for All, described as "a national health plan . . . in which all Americans would get their insurance from a single government plan." A majority of Americans supported Medicare for All in all fifteen polls.[61]

Experts are analyzing the merits of the policy. Pundits are debating its chances in our politics. But one thing has become clear: it's time to take Medicare for All seriously.

PART II

POLICY

3

MEDICARE FOR ALL

THE FUNDAMENTALS

The architects of Medicare always intended the program to be a first step toward universal national health insurance. But healthcare in the United States has evolved considerably since Medicare was first enacted in 1965. What would it look like to bring Medicare to all Americans in the twenty-first century?

In Part II of this book, we dissect Medicare for All as a policy. In this chapter we outline the core features of Medicare for All (M4A) and evaluate how M4A would address the major problems in the US healthcare system. In Chapter 4 we take a deep dive into the major choices that must be made in the design and implementation of M4A. In Chapter 5 we examine how to pay for M4A, and in Chapter 6 we evaluate how M4A compares to alternative health reform proposals.

WHAT IS MEDICARE FOR ALL?

Medicare for All is a proposal to create a single, publicly funded insurance plan that provides comprehensive healthcare coverage to all Americans. M4A would be an American version of a single-payer health insurance system, with one payer (Medicare) funding healthcare for the entire population.

M4A would be an enhanced version of the traditional Medicare program that tens of millions of seniors rely on today. Other Americans would transition from their current insurance to M4A, including people who have employer-based insurance, Medicaid, or private Medicare Advantage plans. People who are currently uninsured would also gain coverage through M4A. Much like Medicare or Social Security today, M4A would not be an opt-in or opt-out program; everyone would be covered.

An important feature is that private hospitals and doctors would remain private under M4A. This distinguishes M4A from "socialized medicine" systems like the Veterans Health Administration in the United States or the National Health Service in the United Kingdom, where the government owns most of the hospitals and employs most clinicians directly. M4A would be more like the Canadian healthcare system, where the payment system is public but the delivery system of doctors and hospitals remains private. In short, M4A would change how we pay for care, not who provides care.

Here's another important clarification: M4A would not simply expand Medicare in its current form to the entire population. Rather, Medicare itself would change. The existing Medicare program has numerous features that M4A proponents seek to do away with. Today's Medicare consists of separate insurance plans for hospital care and physician services (a legacy of the legislative maneuvering described in Chapter 2), and prescription drug coverage must be purchased separately from a private company. Major benefit categories are left out, including vision, dental, hearing, and long-term care. Hospital insurance is financed through taxes, but beneficiaries must pay a separate premium for physician insurance and drug coverage. Patients also face high out-of-pocket costs. Medicare's physician insurance only covers 80 percent of costs, and Medicare's hospital insurance is literally a high-deductible health plan.[1] Because of these gaps in coverage, most Medicare beneficiaries carry yet another insurance plan (a supplementary or Medigap plan) to round out their coverage.

Furthermore, a third of seniors choose to exit the traditional Medicare plan altogether, instead opting for a Medicare Advantage plan managed by a private insurance company. Medicare Advantage plans appeal to seniors by offering reduced out-of-pocket costs or extra benefits like vision and dental; in exchange, plans restrict access to providers and put tighter controls on the use of care.

The bottom line is that M4A proponents seek to improve and expand Medicare, not sign all Americans up for the current system. In Chapters 4 and 5, we'll consider a series of important questions that legislators and the public must face when spelling out the details of a Medicare for All program. Will private insurance companies have *any* role in this system? Exactly which services are covered by M4A, and which are free at the point of use? How are doctors paid, and how much? How is the system funded? These choices have trade-offs we'll discuss in those chapters. But in this chapter we'll focus on the more fundamental question of how M4A would change American healthcare as a whole.

THE ACTIVE INGREDIENTS OF M4A

There are six "active ingredients" that make M4A work: universal coverage, comprehensive coverage, pricing power, administrative efficiency, progressive financing, and public accountability. M4A would achieve universal coverage, but the changes envisioned by M4A are broader and deeper than that basic fact. After all, even those who have insurance in today's system often lack access to the healthcare they need, or they end up paying dearly for it. Under M4A, coverage would become not just universal but comprehensive. Costs would be controlled because M4A has both pricing power and administrative efficiency. Because health insurance would move from the private sector to the public sector, M4A would make healthcare financing more progressive, and health insurance would become publicly accountable. We'll examine each of these active ingredients in turn, then consider how they help M4A address the problems in American healthcare.

Universal Coverage

This one is simple: Medicare for All guarantees healthcare coverage to every American. Though there may be political battles over including undocumented Americans (as we'll discuss in Chapter 4), M4A legislation in the 2019–20 Congress proposed to cover "every individual who is a resident of the United States." Uninsurance in the United States would be essentially eliminated.

Furthermore, coverage under M4A would be secure. In today's precarious system, Americans can lose their health insurance for any number of reasons: losing a job, getting a new job, moving to a different state, turning in paperwork late, losing a parent, losing a spouse, divorcing a spouse, giving birth, turning nineteen, turning twenty-six, getting work hours cut, or getting a raise. Under M4A, every American would have secure, lifelong health coverage no matter how their circumstances might change.

Comprehensive Coverage

Medicare for All also seeks to make Americans' health coverage comprehensive. Leading proposals for Medicare for All would cover a full range of benefits with minimal or no out-of-pocket costs. People could get their care from any participating clinician or hospital and would no longer need to worry about surprise bills for out-of-network services.

These would be significant changes for the vast majority of Americans, alleviating the gaps in access we detailed in Chapter 1. Medicare for All seeks to return health coverage to its core purpose: to make sure that every person can get the care they need to stay well and the treatment they need when they're sick, and to make sure the costs are covered.

Medicare for All would also expand Americans' choice of doctors and hospitals. All participating providers would be considered in-network for all Americans. And because alternatives to M4A would be limited, participation of providers would be virtually guaranteed. Indeed, almost all physicians accept Medicare today, even though it only covers about a fifth of the population. Just 2 percent of primary care physicians don't accept Medicare patients, compared to 4 percent who don't accept patients with private insurance (and 32 percent who don't accept Medicaid patients).[2] All told, in a country with nearly 1 million physicians, around 25,000 have opted out of Medicare—about 2.5 percent.[3] In essence, Medicare for All would trade the choice of insurance plan for the choice of doctor and hospital.

Pricing Power

By insuring all Americans, M4A becomes a monopsony in healthcare. This is different from a monopoly, where there's only one seller of a good; in a monopsony there's only one *buyer* of a good. That gives the single buyer considerable negotiating leverage, which Medicare could use to rein in the cost of drugs, hospital stays, and physician services.

High prices are a leading cause of high healthcare spending in the United States, and prices in the private insurance system are currently determined by business negotiations between individual insurance companies and healthcare providers. Our fragmented system leaves insurance companies with limited leverage in these negotiations, allowing drug companies and healthcare providers to charge high and rising prices. Insurance companies also face perverse incentives that encourage them to keep prices high in many cases. In contrast, the current Medicare program uses its leverage to set lower prices that keep costs under control.

Physicians negotiate prices with private insurers that are about 40 percent higher on average than they receive from Medicare (with a smaller markup for primary care and a larger markup for specialized services and procedures.)[4] Hospitals, meanwhile, negotiate prices with private insurers that are *double* Medicare rates on average.[5] It's no surprise that when Americans with private insurance turn 65 and switch to Medicare, their spending drops precipitously due to lower prices.[6] By extending Medicare's negotiating power to all Americans, M4A would be a powerful mechanism to keep prices in check across the entire healthcare system.

There are trade-offs to determining payment rates through public regulation instead of private negotiations. Economists generally believe that when markets function perfectly, the forces of supply and demand lead to prices that reflect the true value of the product being sold, and that government regulation of prices tends to interfere with this process. But as detailed in Chapter 1, healthcare does not function like a normal market good. In a system where the price of a basic service like an MRI can vary by a factor of four within the same city, where drug patents make competition illegal, and where 90 percent of hospital markets are highly concentrated, it is difficult to argue that private sector prices are the result of a well-functioning marketplace settling on the true value of services. On a more fundamental level, patients simply do not act like consumers in the traditional sense—we lack full information, are shielded from the full price tag by insurance, need to make decisions quickly or under duress, and often have no real alternative to getting treatment when and where we need it. Price regulation is premised on the argument that the consumer choice model of healthcare has failed to deliver on its promise.

Public sector regulation of payment rates will never be perfect. Regulators make decisions using imperfect information, the regulatory process takes time to complete, and the process is subject to lobbying. Nevertheless, Medicare has over thirty years of experience setting payment rates and has had better success in controlling medical spending relative to the private sector.

Administrative Efficiency

Private insurance companies incur overhead costs five times greater than Medicare does, and in turn the fragmented private insurance system imposes considerable costs on clinicians and hospitals, who must interact with a staggering array of insurance plans.[7] High administrative costs are the second leading cause of high US healthcare spending, and M4A could save hundreds of billions of dollars annually by transitioning to a single public insurer. The administrative simplicity of a single payer would also decrease the time that clinicians and patients spend dealing with insurance issues.

Progressive Financing

Private health insurance is financed regressively, with low-income families spending three times as much of their income on healthcare compared to high-income families[8] (*Regressive* means low-income people pay more relative to their income; *progressive* means high-income people pay more.) That's because the rich, the poor, and the middle-class face the same employer-sponsored insurance premiums, which can be an enormous burden for poor families, yet a relatively minor expense for wealthy families. The tax break for job-based insurance makes the system even more regressive, with the greatest benefit going to people in the highest tax brackets. High out-of-pocket costs are also a regressive strategy for financing healthcare: a $2,400 deductible might be a minor inconvenience for an investment banker but a month's salary for a bank teller. M4A could replace the regressive financing of private insurance with progressive taxation, saving money for middle-class and low-income families.

Progressive financing of healthcare is a question not just of economics but of values. Consumer products are usually paid for regressively, with people of all income levels facing the same out-of-pocket cost for a given automobile, restaurant, or iPhone—even if that means poorer families pay a larger percentage of income. In contrast, many people believe we should pay for public goods using progressive taxes. For instance, instead of funding the US military with a $2,300 fee on every person in America (which is the per-person cost of our military budget), the federal government raises the revenue using progressive taxes. Similarly, we don't charge every family a fixed tuition to send their child to a public elementary school; we expect richer families to chip in relatively more through property taxes. When it comes to health insurance, progressive financing is part of the broader ethical vision of treating healthcare not as a consumer product but as a public good.[9]

Public Accountability

For-profit insurance companies are ultimately accountable to their shareholders. Because of this, private insurers are incentivized to behave in ways that enhance profits, even if this contradicts the best interests of the public's health—for instance, selectively enrolling healthy patients, or erecting barriers to care for patients who require expensive treatment. Profit-oriented companies often abandon initiatives that improve health if they don't also come with a financial return on investment. In contrast, M4A would be accountable to the American public. Like Medicare today, constraints on spending under M4A might emerge from concern about the government budget or the deficit, and in turn the burden on current and future taxpayers. But unlike a for-profit company, M4A can justify its decisions based on public health benefit and social mission rather than cost-cutting or profit-making.

Some are critical of the fact that M4A would create a larger role for government in making decisions about health coverage. These critics argue that our political system is hyperpartisan, susceptible to gridlock, marred by corruption, and unduly influenced by powerful corporations and other special interests. Furthermore, in an era of political polarization, Democrats who support single-payer healthcare in principle might worry about what would happen to M4A under a Republican president, and likewise Republicans might chafe at the thought of a Democratic administration making decisions about their family's health coverage.

The resilience of the existing Medicare program quells many of these hypothetical concerns. Since its passage in 1965, Medicare has persisted through more than fifty sessions of Congress, including periods of unified control by both Democrats and Republicans. Medicare has also persisted through ten presidential administrations, including leaders as ideologically diverse as Jimmy Carter, Ronald Reagan, Barack Obama, and Donald Trump. Nevertheless, Medicare remains a strong program that Americans of all stripes can rely on. Neither political party is eager to undermine a universal program that Americans of all backgrounds depend on.

Furthermore, public accountability for health insurance must be compared to the alternative: control by large, increasingly consolidated insurance corporations that are ultimately accountable to shareholders rather than the public.

Those are the active ingredients of Medicare for All: universal coverage, comprehensive coverage, pricing power, administrative efficiency, progressive financing, and public accountability. Given these elements, how would M4A address the major problems in American healthcare? In Chapter 1 we established that the four key problems facing the US healthcare system are that it is too expensive, too few people have access to it, it doesn't do enough to improve our health, and it is eroding the experience of giving and receiving care. Let's now examine how M4A might address each of these four problems.

PROBLEM #1: OUR HEALTHCARE IS TOO EXPENSIVE

Medicare for All has the potential to make healthcare more affordable because it addresses three critical sources of high spending: prices charged by hospitals and doctors, administrative costs, and drug prices.

"It's the Prices, Stupid"

Remember the first major driver of our high healthcare spending: high prices. Compared to people in other countries, Americans don't use more prescription drugs, spend more time in the hospital, or see the doctor more often. But Americans are charged far more every time they do need any of these things.

Our prices are so high because even though healthcare doesn't work like a normal market good, we still buy and sell it in a private marketplace. This allows hospitals, doctors, imaging centers, emergency departments, and ambulance companies to charge the highest prices in the world—and neither individual patients nor our fragmented system of private insurers has the power to stop them. This problem has been exacerbated by a torrent of mergers that has reshaped the healthcare system into a patchwork of local monopolies and oligopolies that have even more power to demand higher prices from privately insured patients.

M4A would neutralize the power of local monopolies, and more generally would prevent providers from taking advantage of a broken marketplace to raise prices. Unlike private insurance companies, M4A would not need to capitulate to the demands of large hospital systems. Like Medicare today, M4A would have the power to directly determine how much it pays for different kinds of care. Because Medicare is such a big program, nearly all doctors and hospitals find it beneficial to accept Medicare's rates, and the same would be true under Medicare for All. Crucially, the savings from enhanced negotiating power do not represent a one-time fix. M4A's negotiating power could keep prices in check indefinitely, which could allow America to finally get a hold on runaway spending growth.

We can see the enormous potential for cost savings by comparing the current Medicare program to our private insurance system. Over the past two decades, hospital prices in private insurance have increased far more rapidly than in Medicare.[10] In terms of overall healthcare spending, between 2008 and 2018 per-person spending by private insurers increased by more than 50 percent, while spending by Medicare increased by about 20 percent.[11] Achieving this slower growth rate systemwide could save trillions of dollars each decade. Though private sector dogma assumes private companies have more tools and greater incentive (via profit motive) to keep spending down, the evidence is clear that Medicare controls spending better than private insurers do. The reason is simple: Medicare has the leverage to keep prices under control, and private insurers don't.

Reducing Administrative Costs

Our complex private insurance system saddles the United States with the highest administrative costs in the world. M4A has the capacity to vastly reduce the amount of money we spend on administration. In 2017, the United States spent $812 billion on healthcare administration—$2,500 for every American.[12] Canada's single-payer system spent just $550 per person. If the United States was able to achieve Canadian levels of administrative spending by moving to a single-payer system, we would save $600 billion per year. These savings are enormous, equivalent to 17 percent of total national health spending in 2017. Even if administrative spending under M4A wasn't reduced all the way to Canadian levels, there is little doubt that the annual savings could total in the hundreds of billions of dollars.

These savings would come from two places: reduced insurance overhead and reduced administrative burden on providers.

Insurance overhead would be reduced immediately. Private insurers incur overhead costs of 13 percent to support redundant administrative functions across each individual corporation, plus marketing costs, multimillion-dollar salaries, and profit.[13] By contrast, in 2018 the traditional Medicare program operated with a 2.3 percent overhead.[14] A Medicare for All program would be expected to perform similarly.[15] This alone could save trillions of dollars each decade.

Hospitals, doctors, nursing homes, and home health agencies would also be relieved of the administrative burden of a fractured payment system. Instead of spending time and money dealing with the arcane requirements of hundreds of different health plans—not just billing, but getting required authorizations from each insurer to provide different services, navigating conflicting lists of covered medications, reporting varying quality metrics to fulfill the requirements of different insurers, and managing constantly evolving networks of specialists, laboratories, and imaging centers—providers could use one streamlined system that would free up resources to focus on clinical care. Unlike for insurance overhead, where Medicare provides a direct comparison, there are no readily available American data to help predict how much providers would save on administration if we moved to a single-payer system. But in Canada's single-payer system, providers spend half as much of their revenue on administration compared to the United States.[16] These savings could also amount to trillions of dollars each decade.

It's worth pausing to understand where these savings fit into the system as a whole. Here's a simple equation we'll revisit in future chapters: *Income = (Price × Quantity) − Operating Costs.* This just means providers make more money if they raise their prices, get reimbursed for more services, or decrease their operating costs. Providers experience the administrative savings of single-payer reform as decreased operating costs; all else equal, this raises their income. But this also means that to some extent, M4A could reduce prices *without* decreasing the incomes of providers—it's simply a way to pass the savings from administrative efficiency to the public.

Lowering the Price of Prescription Drugs

Negotiating on behalf of hundreds of millions of Americans, M4A would have considerable power to bring down prices for prescription drugs. Similar to the way that M4A neutralizes the power of large hospital systems, M4A would shift the balance of power away from drug companies and toward the public.

Drug price negotiation is not a foreign idea. The US Department of Veterans Affairs negotiates drug prices, and as a result it secures prices approximately 40 percent lower than the prices paid by Medicare.[17] In Chapter 4 we explore more fully how this negotiation could work and what the impact would be on the production of innovative drugs. But there's no question that M4A could significantly reduce drug prices.

Because our healthcare system is so complex, it can be easy to forget that one basic structural feature drives so much of our high spending: the decision to rely on a large number of private companies to both set medical prices and administer insurance benefits. Reducing the panoply of private insurance companies to a single public insurer would tackle our major cost drivers in one fell swoop.

The Costs—and Who Bears Them

Of course, M4A would also increase healthcare spending in important ways: covering the Americans who are currently uninsured, reducing out-of-pocket costs, and providing more comprehensive benefits to virtually all Americans. In Chapter 5 we outline how experts tally up the costs and savings of M4A. Unsurprisingly, the devil is in the details—and the details matter to the tune of trillions of dollars. But in very rough terms, the new costs of expanded coverage under M4A are likely to be similar in size to the savings from administrative costs, drug prices, and provider payment rates. And because M4A has more powerful tools to slow cost growth, M4A is likely to cost less than our current system over time.

PROBLEM #2: TOO MANY AMERICANS STILL CAN'T ACCESS HEALTHCARE

Americans currently experience five major barriers to medical care. First, many Americans have no health coverage at all. Second, many Americans with insurance still face large financial barriers to care because they cannot afford their copays or deductibles. Third, many Americans get turned away from care because doctors reject their insurance, or their insurance doesn't cover all the services they need. Fourth, many Americans simply lack the doctors and hospitals in their community to get the care they need. Fifth and finally, Americans who enjoy adequate healthcare today cannot be sure it will still be there when they need it. M4A would help alleviate each of these barriers.

Under Medicare for All, everyone would have guaranteed healthcare coverage from the day they are born until the day they die. As detailed in Chapter 4, M4A could be designed to eliminate or vastly reduce out-of-pocket costs for medically necessary care.

Under M4A, there would be no restricted or narrow networks, and no surprise out-of-network bills. Americans would be free to choose whatever doctor they prefer. While every American could benefit from increased choice of provider, the difference would be particularly meaningful for Medicaid patients. Doctors (including primary care physicians) currently turn away Medicaid patients at higher rates, because they are paid less for treating Medicaid patients. By building equity into our payment policy, M4A would end the system where low-income Americans are treated as second-class healthcare citizens.

M4A could also improve access to healthcare in rural communities. Hospitals in poor rural areas are shutting down at alarming rates, and our health insurance system is partly to blame: in addition to having a lower volume of patients to begin with, rural hospitals treat large numbers of uninsured patients, Medicaid patients, and underinsured patients who can't afford their bills. Under M4A, every rural American would have comprehensive health coverage and hospitals would no longer get paid less for treating poorer patients. These changes could help these critical hospitals remain financially solvent, stemming the tide of rural hospital closures. This helps people in rural communities access critical medical services, and also protects rural economies because hospitals often serve as one of the largest employers in these communities.

Finally, M4A would make American healthcare more resilient. The Great Recession and the COVID-19 pandemic both exposed a painful feature of our healthcare system: an economic downturn is liable to throw millions of Americans off their health coverage. Instead of protecting people during times of crisis, our health insurance system makes those crises worse. And even in normal times, Americans live under the constant threat of losing their private health insurance if they lose their job, or losing Medicaid if they get a raise or move to a different state, or losing their coverage for any other reason as they struggle to navigate our precarious and fragmented system. Under M4A, Americans would no longer face the insecurity of losing their health insurance when personal or economic circumstances change.

Furthermore, the COVID-19 pandemic revealed that our healthcare institutions are themselves precarious. With elective surgeries cancelled and many Americans avoiding care altogether during the pandemic, the United States faced an absurd and tragic reality: many of our hospitals and health centers were on the brink of financial collapse when they were needed most. This partly reflects the fact that American healthcare institutions are primarily funded like businesses—and like other businesses, they suffered when their most lucrative customers stayed home. Financial losses were exacerbated because millions of Americans who lost their jobs went onto Medicaid—which pays providers much less than private insurance—or became completely uninsured, all of which meant less revenue to keep our healthcare system afloat during the pandemic. Under M4A, every American would maintain their health coverage during a crisis, which would stabilize both individual families and the healthcare system as a whole. And as discussed further in Chapter 4, M4A could change the way that we pay providers to keep their funding stable even when economic conditions change.

In sum, M4A seeks to give all Americans reliable access to healthcare no matter their life circumstances—and to make the healthcare system itself more resilient.

PROBLEM #3: AMERICANS ARE SICKER THAN OUR PEERS

Tackling Severe Illness among the Poor and Marginalized

Our unequal society leads to especially severe illness among marginalized communities. Many causes of illness lie outside the medical system. But instead of fighting inequality, our current healthcare system exacerbates it.

In the current American system, the quality of healthcare received depends importantly on race and socioeconomic status, and our health insurance system is one driver of these disparities—the uninsured and underinsured are disproportionately low-income and people of color. Poor and non-white Americans are left with poorer access to healthcare. M4A would provide *all* Americans quality coverage, regardless of income or race.

Lower-income Americans are also kept away from care through high out-of-pocket costs. The average private health insurance plan has a deductible in the thousands of dollars, but nearly half of adults with health insurance say they don't have enough readily accessible savings to cover an unexpected $500 expense.[18] It's no surprise that lower-income Americans are more likely to avoid necessary care because of cost. By reducing or eliminating out-of-pocket costs, M4A would let all Americans access the care they need, without discriminating based on income. And the evidence is clear: Americans are healthier and live longer when they have better access to healthcare. By covering the uninsured, Medicare for All could save tens of thousands of lives every year.[19]

Economic deprivation is another important driver of poor health. Our healthcare system contributes to economic deprivation by driving millions of people into poverty, both because overall costs are high and because low-income employer-insured families are charged the same high prices as the wealthy.[20] By making healthcare financing more progressive, M4A doubles as an antipoverty program. The comprehensive coverage provided by M4A would also protect against the financial toxicity of illness and help end the specter of medical bankruptcy. Furthermore, we know that better health insurance has spillover benefits to the broader material conditions of a person's life, including financial health, housing stability, food security, and stable employment—all of which loop back to improve health in the long term.

In short, in today's America being sick can make you poor, and being poor can make you sick. M4A could help break this cycle.

Wellness, Public Health, and Social Services

Public health experts generally believe that as a society, the United States should invest more in wellness than we currently do. M4A has the potential to address a major barrier to that: our healthcare payment system.

One problem with the current payment system is "churn" across insurance plans, which discourages investment in prevention and wellness. As a society, we *want* to invest in measures that prevent heart attacks, joint problems, and cancer ten or twenty years in the future. But almost no one keeps the same insurance plan for ten or twenty years. When you change jobs, you change insurance plans. If you lose your job, you might go onto Medicaid, only to come off when you get another job. When your employer signs a new insurance contract, you change plans. Every year you can buy a different plan in the ACA marketplace. This system of endless hopping between insurance plans is a major roadblock for incentivizing prevention because every insurer knows that their investments will likely end up accruing value for a different insurer at the end of the day—often to Medicare, which insures every American over sixty-five. Churn is a problem not just for preventive measures but also for expensive therapies like hepatitis C treatment, where the potential complications averted by early treatment (such as liver cancer) might occur decades in the future, giving insurance companies less incentive to pay the up-front cost.

More fundamentally, a hard truth of health policy is that investing in prevention is the right thing to do, but it often doesn't save money. After all, many people need to receive a preventive service to avoid one expensive outcome down the line—for example, on average 100 people need to take blood pressure medications for five years to prevent a heart attack in one person.[21] This presents a problem when payment decisions are made by for-profit insurance companies: initiatives that improve health but decrease profits might be left on the cutting room floor.

Because M4A would cover people from birth till death, it would solve the problem of churn. Instead of jumping from plan to plan every few years, Americans would stay with M4A for life. This incentivizes long-term investments in prevention. The American public would make the investments, and the American public would benefit from them. And on a more fundamental level, M4A has more freedom to act like a public health program rather than a business, making investments that improve health but *don't* benefit the bottom line.

A unified payment system also gives M4A more power to align medical payments with social needs. One of the largest opportunities for reform is in primary care. Primary care providers tend to be underpaid relative to their specialist counterparts. By bolstering reimbursements for primary care, M4A would have the power to increase the number of primary care doctors over time by making this critically important profession a more attractive career choice. This is just one example of the public health goals that can be pursued by a national payer beholden to the public rather than shareholders.

Furthermore, in many countries, medical care, public health, and social services all draw from the same budget. This allows for a more thoughtful allocation of resources across these different sectors—and it's most likely better for overall health to put relatively more of the budget into public health and social services that improve the conditions of life instead of medical care that only takes care of you after you have gotten sick. To be sure, moving to M4A would not automatically lead to increased investments in public health and social services. But by shifting health insurance into the public sector and covering Americans across the life span, M4A might open up the opportunity to coordinate healthcare spending and broader social investments in a more intentional way.

The point of public health and social services is not to save money—it's to improve the quality of life in a society. Nevertheless, the case for investment in public health and social services is stronger if the government will experience some of the savings from averted medical expenses.

PROBLEM #4: THE EXPERIENCE OF GIVING AND RECEIVING CARE IS ERODING

One of the biggest challenges in the health system is that consolidation, complexity, and a heightened focus on the financial elements of medicine have eroded the experience of care for patients as well as doctors, nurses, and other medical staff.

One way that M4A could help is by slowing the tide of consolidation in healthcare. One driver of healthcare mergers is the fact that our private insurance system rewards providers with higher fees when they merge and increase their bargaining leverage against insurers. Under a Medicare for All payment system, consolidated providers would no longer be able to demand higher fees—removing one of the most important (and perverse) incentives for corporate consolidation in healthcare. Still, the ability to leverage higher payment rates is only one driver of consolidation. To fully combat this trend, M4A would need to be combined with traditional antitrust tools, putting heightened scrutiny on mergers and other anticompetitive behavior by both for-profit and non-profit provider groups.

Medicare for All would also contribute to an improved experience of care by simplifying the onerous administrative tasks currently faced by both patients and clinicians, and by reducing the constant intrusion of financial considerations between doctors and patients.

Empowering Doctors

The incentives that drive healthcare systems to get bigger and bigger have spurred them to buy up doctors' practices at increasing rates. With enormous hospital systems dominating the market—and reaping the increased revenue from their monopoly power—small, independent practices are left at a serious competitive disadvantage.[22] Under M4A, many doctors would still work for large systems, but other physicians could capitalize on the freedom to practice in other settings without facing a major financial disadvantage.

M4A's unified payment system also means that physicians would be able to treat all patients equally. The current system penalizes physicians for caring for Medicaid patients through low reimbursement rates. M4A would embed equality into the structure of the payment system, which would transform care for the poor from an act of charity into a normal function of an equitable health system.

The administrative simplification of M4A would also free up clinician time to focus on patient care. Physicians today spend too much of their time jumping through administrative hoops to satisfy the requirements of insurance companies. The electronic medical record, the way we manage the reams of patient data online, is one current scapegoat of this administrative burden. Indeed, for every hour that a physician spends with a patient, they spend two hours doing computer work.[23] One revealing study showed that doctors' notes in the electronic medical record are four times longer in America than they are in other countries—even when foreign doctors use the *exact same software* as American doctors. Why? The sheer complexity of our billing system appears to play a large role. The researchers found that in other countries, a doctor's note tends to contain "only essential clinical information; it omits much of the compliance and reimbursement documentation that commonly bloats the American clinical note."[24] M4A could mean less time on computer work and less time on the phone with insurance companies—and more time with patients.

Empowering Nurses and Other Staff

Nurses and clinical support staff spend more time with patients than any other category of provider in the hospital. However, they have been largely squeezed by the consolidation that has occurred over the past several decades. M4A could help empower nurses and other staff by slowing down provider consolidation and preserving the viability of independent practices; with more employment options, healthcare workers have greater protection from the harmful practices of dominant employers. This could also give healthcare employees more power to secure workers' rights and safe staffing practices, and could bolster the ability of unions to stand up to employers. As with doctors, simplifying our insurance system would also allow nurses to shift their time away from administrative tasks and toward patient care.

The Experience of Care

Medicare for All could help make clinical encounters feel less like a financial transaction and more like a healing provider-patient relationship. Our current system exacts a large toll on the time and psyche of patients who need to spend their most vulnerable moments deciphering medical bills, arguing with insurance companies, and worrying whether they will be able to pay for recommended treatments. On the other end of the encounter, doctors and nurses face the constant frustration of knowing they're failing their patients because of holes in our healthcare system that are out of their control. At its best, Medicare for All offers an opportunity to help restore healthcare's focus on care and healing.

The American healthcare system is too expensive, leaves too many without access to care, falls short in improving our health, and damages the experience of clinicians and patients. Medicare for All seeks to tackle these problems by bringing all Americans into the system with universal and comprehensive coverage, saving money by simplifying administration and reining in prices, shifting costs away from the middle class and the poor through progressive financing, and making the system more accountable to the public.

On the most fundamental level, Medicare for All seeks to transform our medical marketplace into a health system where care is guaranteed to all.

4

DESIGNING A MEDICARE FOR ALL PROGRAM

Medicare for All is a very simple idea: establish a comprehensive, publicly financed insurance program that covers all Americans. But translating that core premise into a final piece of legislation—and then turning that legislation into an actual functioning program—will require dozens of consequential policy decisions. Many of these decisions might appear to be technical. But in fact, almost all of them flow from a deeper question about which values the American public wants to write into their healthcare system. Health is, after all, the least common denominator, and healthcare is an intimate mirror of our social and political values. Who gets it? How much do they get? What does it cover? How much has to be paid by the recipient? Answers to all of these questions will come to reflect deeply held values.

These policy questions will also shape the political debate around Medicare for All. In the words of Princeton economist Uwe Reinhardt, "Every dollar of healthcare spending is someone else's dollar of healthcare income, including fraud, waste, and abuse." When Medicare for All legislation affects how hospitals, physicians, and drug companies get paid, these groups will naturally have an intense political interest in the outcome. This is even more true for private insurance companies, whose entire business model is threatened by Medicare for All.

On the flip side, the design of Medicare for All will also shape popular support for the policy. If the coverage offered by Medicare for All is viewed by most Americans as being no better than what they currently have, there is little hope for building a popular movement for its passage.

And there's no free lunch in healthcare. Policy choices that make Medicare for All more expensive—adding more benefits, minimizing out-of-pocket costs, paying hospitals and drug companies more generously—will need to be paid for on the back end.

At the time of writing, there are two Medicare for All bills in the US Congress (116th Congress, 2019–20). The House bill is HR1384, sponsored by Representative Pramila Jayapal from Washington's Seventh Congressional District. The Senate bill is S1129, sponsored by Senator Bernie Sanders from Vermont. Throughout this chapter we will refer to these bills to give a point-in-time snapshot of how congressional legislation aims to resolve the policy questions we outline.

This chapter outlines the critical choices that policymakers designing a Medicare for All system will face. As the debate about M4A continues in the public discourse, and as M4A legislation moves through the legislative process, these key questions will arise again and again. Here we detail seven of the most important policy questions and describe the major policy options on the table to answer them. We then analyze some major strengths and weaknesses involved in each. This chapter, then, serves as a guide to the M4A policy debate.

QUESTION #1: WHAT BENEFITS ARE COVERED, AND FOR WHOM?

A core tenet of M4A is establishing a program that covers a *comprehensive* set of services. But which services would be included, exactly?

There's consensus that Medicare for All would cover at least the basic services covered by both Medicare and private insurance today: for instance, physician services, hospital care, mental health and addiction services, prescription drugs, and emergency services. The more relevant question is what services M4A would add, over and above what Medicare already covers. Both S1129 and HR1384 propose to add coverage for dental, vision, and hearing—services that many Americans lack today, particularly seniors, given that the current Medicare program does not offer coverage.

One significant question is whether M4A would add coverage for long-term services and supports. Long-term care services are used by people of all ages who need assistance to perform routine daily activities, generally due to aging, disability, or chronic illness. These services are increasingly provided in a person's own home or in community-based programs. When necessary, long-term care can also be provided in nursing homes or other institutions.

For many Americans, long-term care is a catastrophic expense. Medicare does not currently cover long-term care, even though current estimates suggest that one in three Americans turning sixty-five will need nursing home care at some point in their lives—not to mention the millions of Americans requiring long-term support within the home, often provided by unpaid caregivers in the family.[1] Nursing home stays can cost up to $100,000 per year, so seniors often rapidly deplete their savings.[2] Eventually seniors' assets are drawn down so drastically that they qualify for Medicaid, which does cover long-term care. In fact, even though Medicaid is known as the insurer for low-income adults and children, two-thirds of Medicaid spending goes toward seniors and people with disabilities. The current system, in many ways, pushes seniors who require long-term care into poverty.

As you might expect, American seniors have been pushing to add long-term care benefits to Medicare since at least the 1980s.[3] Covering long-term services and supports under M4A would be a marked improvement for the significant portion of Americans who will require these services at some point in their lives.

Long-term care is expensive. Depending on the nature of the benefit, long-term care could add hundreds of billions of dollars to the annual costs of M4A—equivalent to about $700 per American per year, according to one estimate.[4] This would represent one of the largest new costs of the program.

A second significant question is how M4A would cover healthcare that has been politicized—services such as comprehensive reproductive care, including abortion, or gender affirmation surgery for trans Americans. Under current law (known as the Hyde Amendment), federal funds cannot be used to pay for abortion. M4A legislation including comprehensive reproductive services would require a repeal of the Hyde Amendment. Though providing these services under M4A is critical to ensuring equitable access to reproductive healthcare, it is likely to be a flash point for debate given the politicization of abortion.

Policymakers will also need to decide *who* is eligible for benefits. Like abortion services, care for undocumented immigrants is likely to be highly politicized. Politicians who favor tighter immigration laws often attack undocumented immigrants as a "drain on the system," particularly when it comes to healthcare use. However, because immigrants are more likely to be young and in the workforce, evidence suggests they pay more into the US healthcare system than they receive in benefits. Even now, immigrants are helping prop up the Medicare program: immigrants overall (both citizens and noncitizens) pay more into the Medicare trust fund than they take out, while US-born Americans actually take more out of the Medicare trust fund than they pay in.[5] Undocumented immigrants are also subsidizing the private insurance system: undocumented immigrants pay more in premiums than they receive in benefits (an excess contribution of $1,400 per person each year), while US-born Americans take more out of the private insurance pool than they pay in premiums.[6] While a common political narrative insists that US-born Americans subsidize healthcare for immigrants, the exact opposite appears to be true. Nevertheless, care for undocumented immigrants under M4A is certain to be politicized.

Beyond broad categories of services, the process by which M4A would decide to cover specific tests, services, and procedures (including those invented after M4A is implemented) would need to be developed. Under the current Medicare program, a service is covered if it is deemed to be "reasonable and necessary." These coverage determinations can be made by Medicare at the national level or by one of its contractors at the local or regional level. These judgments about what is "reasonable and necessary" generally do not consider either the cost of a service or its comparative effectiveness relative to other options. M4A could build on this current system, or it could add additional requirements for a service to qualify for coverage. M4A would also need to specify whether certain covered services require patients to get a referral in advance. Though granular, these kinds of details will have an important influence on the day-to-day experience of the program.

QUESTION #2: HOW MUCH COMES OUT OF POCKET, AND FOR WHAT SERVICES?

Some public services require a fee for every use, like taking a city bus or registering a car. But many public services are free at the point of use, like driving on a local street, going to a local park, or calling the fire department to your home.

Should healthcare services provided by Medicare for All—like seeing a doctor or filling a prescription—require beneficiaries to pay at the point of care?

Fees at the point of care come in three main forms. *Deductibles* are the amount you need to spend in a year before insurance kicks in at all. *Copayments* are fixed fees you pay with every use of a service. And *coinsurance* is a percentage of the cost that you're asked to cover. Collectively, these payments are known as "cost-sharing"—the insurance company shares the cost with you, the patient.

Many economists argue that health insurance should include out-of-pocket fees at the point of care. The argument for cost-sharing is based on the idea of "moral hazard." To illustrate: If you own a car but don't have car insurance, you'll probably be *very* careful not to damage your car, because fixing it will be very expensive. But if you have car insurance that fully covers the cost of repairs, you'll be less careful with the car—meaning you'll get into more accidents, and you'll generally have a lower threshold to come into the shop for fixes. Essentially, moral hazard is the propensity to use more services than you need if you don't have to pay for them out of pocket.

Researchers have spent decades studying and debating cost-sharing in healthcare. The basic finding is clear: people use less healthcare if you make them pay more for it. The question is *what* healthcare they use less of. Are people cutting back only on superfluous care that doesn't make them healthier, or are they forgoing appropriate medical treatment that does?

The research is also quite clear on this issue: cost-sharing tends to reduce healthcare use *across the board.*[7] In other words, when patients are faced with high out-of-pocket costs, they do not become "smart shoppers" who pay for exactly the care they need and no more. They simply get less healthcare of all kinds. After all, when it comes to healthcare, most people use it—all of it—because they think it will make them healthier.

For example, one excellent study examined what happened when a large employer forced all its workers to switch from a plan with no cost-sharing into a high-deductible plan.[8] Healthcare spending went down by over 12 percent across the board. But workers did *not* price-shop to find better deals, and they did not substitute less expensive care for more expensive care. They simply used less care of *all* kinds, including potentially low-value care (e.g., imaging for back pain) as well as high-value care (e.g., colonoscopies and medication for diabetes). Diabetes drugs, for instance, can be highly effective—but the high-deductible plan cut their use in *half.*

Another worrying example of this phenomenon comes from a study of women who underwent a mandated switch into a high-deductible health plan. Even though breast cancer screenings were generally free, women forced into a high-deductible health plan who went on to develop breast cancer had significant delays in their care: they faced delays in receiving diagnostic breast imaging, breast biopsy, and cancer diagnosis. Ultimately, women forced into a high-deductible plan started chemotherapy a full nine months later than their counterparts.[9]

Contrary to the hopes of some proponents, high deductibles don't lead to a more efficient use of healthcare. They simply cut healthcare use across the board.

It is clear that cost-sharing prevents people from getting appropriate medical care. Still, some skeptics question whether this lack of care has a discernible effect on people's health. One classic study in this area is the RAND Health Insurance Experiment, an experiment conducted in the 1970s that randomly assigned people to insurance plans with different levels of cost-sharing. For many patients, the out-of-pocket costs had no measurable impact on health. But the researchers found that low-income patients with hypertension assigned to plans with cost-sharing had worse control of their blood pressure, corresponding to an approximately 10 percent increase in the risk of death.[10] Of course, modern medicine has far more effective therapies to offer for chronic diseases compared to those available in the 1970s, from cancer to heart disease to HIV to opioid addiction. No randomized studies have been conducted in the modern era that specifically assess the overall relationship between cost-sharing and health. But we know that cost-sharing can lead to worse health for some groups of patients, and there is convincing evidence that cost-sharing reduces appropriate medical care of all kinds. Beyond the financial consequences of cost-sharing, these findings about the health consequences are likely to be invoked in the M4A debate.

The issues are similar for prescription drug copays. Unsurprisingly, requiring patients to pay out of pocket for drugs makes them less likely to take the drug. And nonadherence to a prescribed medication regimen is a widespread problem: in a given year, nearly one in three Americans reports not taking their medication as prescribed due to cost.[11]

When it comes to medication, financial barriers can have a real impact on health outcomes. One randomized trial assessed the impact of a copay on taking preventive medications after a heart attack. As expected, patients with copays had a harder time keeping up with their prescribed medication. Significantly, copays also led to worse health outcomes: patients required to pay out of pocket for medications had higher rates of stroke.[12] Moreover, the cost of providing the medications for free was offset by the savings from reduced complications. This is the medical version of a win-win: patients saved money and stayed healthier, at no additional cost to the health system. Other studies have found similar results for different health conditions. For instance, increased out-of-pocket costs for diabetes medications led to decreased adherence, increased hospitalizations, and increased overall healthcare costs.[13]

Value-Based Insurance Design

Some experts have advocated for a middle ground between high deductibles and free care: eliminate out-of-pocket costs, but only for some services and some patients. The idea is to use cost-sharing to nudge people toward valuable care and away from superfluous care. When the *New York Times* interviewed twelve health policy experts about designing a Medicare for All system, several of them advocated for this kind of "value-based" approach to cost-sharing.[14]

The value-based approach would recommend making effective preventive services free. Indeed, there's good evidence that people use more preventive care when it's free, including breast cancer screenings, blood pressure checks, cholesterol checks, and flu vaccinations.[15]

One challenge with this approach is that high deductibles reduce the use of preventive services—even when the preventive services are free![16] Similarly, increased cost-sharing for curative care has been found to decrease the use of preventive care.[17] Though this may seem perplexing, there are multiple possible explanations: patients may not understand the nuances of their highly complex insurance products, high out-of-pocket costs may lead patients to seek care less often in general, or patients are rightly concerned that "free" preventive services could lead to costly interventions down the line (e.g., a screening colonoscopy leading to a polyp removal, or a mammogram requiring a diagnostic biopsy). When healthcare is viewed as a long-term project based on relationships—rather than a set of discrete products purchased at a moment in time—the limitations of these "value-based" nudges come into focus.

Another possibility is a Medicare for All program that eliminates out-of-pocket costs for low-income people but keeps out-of-pocket costs for the middle class and the wealthy. There is certainly a logic to this approach, given that the poor are the most clearly harmed by high out-of-pocket costs. But significant out-of-pocket costs for the middle class and the wealthy also come with trade-offs. High deductibles can dissuade people at all income levels from obtaining appropriate care. In addition, there is an administrative cost to tracking every person's income to determine how much they need to pay each time they step foot in a doctor's office. Politically, there is also an appeal to having a program in which benefits are equal for everyone. Furthermore, reduced out-of-pocket costs for the middle class would likely be an important political selling point for M4A.

In summary, there's a decades-long school of thought in health policy arguing that cost-sharing will nudge patients into choosing "more efficient" care. But a growing body of convincing evidence suggests that cost-sharing simply decreases healthcare use across the board—sometimes to the detriment of patients and the healthcare system writ large.

When it comes to M4A, eliminating out-of-pocket costs would likely increase the use of appropriate medical care. It's also likely to increase the use of low-value care, and to increase healthcare spending overall. For legislators seeking to reduce the costs of M4A, increased cost-sharing is likely to be one of the main policy levers put on the table.

QUESTION #3: WHAT'S THE ROLE FOR PRIVATE INSURANCE?

Under M4A, every American would be covered by Medicare. But that still leaves open the question of what role, if any, private insurance would continue to play.

Public education provides a useful analogy here. Every child in America has the right to an education in a public school. But that leaves open many possible roles for private education: charter schools, private schools, homeschooling, private tutoring, and so forth.

Under a Medicare for All system, what role should private insurance play? There are two major possibilities: private insurance could either supplement or duplicate Medicare.

Supplementing Medicare: Wrap-Around Insurance

In the education system, students in public schools can supplement their studies with private tutoring or other extracurricular enrichment. This is analogous to supplemental health insurance: the public insurance system provides coverage to everyone, and individuals are free to purchase extra private coverage on top. Supplemental private insurance could cover benefits not included under M4A, or it could cover out-of-pocket costs associated with M4A.

Many countries with national health insurance also have a system of supplemental private insurance. Both S1129 (sponsored by Senator Sanders) and HR1384 (sponsored by Representative Jayapal) would allow supplemental private insurance—as does the existing Medicare program, as described later in this chapter.

When it comes to supplemental insurance, the key question is how generous the M4A program itself is—and therefore how much need there is for a supplemental insurance package. If M4A leaves out major categories of care like dental, vision, and prescription drugs, then supplemental insurance is likely to become an important part of the system. If M4A is fully comprehensive, then supplemental insurance is likely to play a very small role, perhaps covering fancier hospital amenities, experimental treatments, or branded prescription drugs when generics are available. In essence, private health insurance would become a luxury product rather than a necessity.

A different kind of supplemental private insurance is a plan that covers out-of-pocket costs. For instance, the current Medicare program requires significant coinsurance payments and has a high deductible; as a result, more than 80 percent of beneficiaries in the traditional Medicare program carry some form of supplemental (Medigap) insurance to cover out-of-pocket expenses.[18] Of course, if M4A had little to no cost-sharing—an issue described in the previous section—there would be no need for private insurance plans that cover out-of-pocket costs. But if a Medicare for All plan was designed with significant cost-sharing, the legislation could allow private plans to cover out-of-pocket expenses. One downside of this setup is that Medigap has particularly high overhead costs: in 2018, more than 21 percent of Medigap premiums were spent on administrative cost and profit.[19] This means that when a senior pays $2,000 a year for a Medigap policy, more than $400 goes toward overhead, marketing, executive salaries, or profit. If the goal is to reduce or eliminate out-of-pocket costs, it's likely more cost-effective to do so directly in the public plan rather than using an additional layer of private insurers.

Duplicating Medicare: Parallel Insurance

In the American education system, everyone pays into the public system, but Americans can choose to pay for a private school instead. This is analogous to duplicative health insurance: everyone pays into the public insurance pool, but people can buy private insurance that operates in parallel to the public program.

Some countries with national health insurance, including the United Kingdom, allow for private insurance that duplicates the public program. These private plans might offer different or faster access to providers. Like the Canadian single-payer system, our current Medicare program does not allow duplicative private insurance; S1129 and HR1384 would also prohibit it.

Proponents of duplicative insurance may argue that it provides a channel to bring additional private funding into the health system rather than relying on taxation, and that the public system would be forced to "compete" with private insurers, perhaps providing an incentive to maintain quality and improve the program over time. Politically, allowing duplicative insurance would also negate the charge that M4A is trying to "ban" private insurance, and it would provide Americans with an additional choice for health coverage.

One drawback of this approach is that duplicative private insurance plans would raise administrative spending, both because the plans themselves would incur significant overhead costs and because they would impose a higher administrative burden on providers. A further risk of duplicative insurance is that some providers could exit the public system or give special priority to privately insured patients, creating a two-tiered system where the wealthy have greater access to care than citizens on the public plan. More generally, public programs are likely to retain broader political support when everyone in society relies on them, rather than the wealthiest and most powerful members of society using their own system.

Replacing Medicare: A Private Option

In the education system, some communities have for-profit charter schools, in effect creating a "private option." When parents choose a for-profit charter school, taxpayer money leaves the public school system and is sent to a private intermediary to deliver a similar service. In health insurance, this is analogous to Medicare Advantage, where taxpayer money is directed out of the public plan and sent to a private company to manage a senior's health insurance benefits. HR1384 and S1129 do not include Medicare Advantage; indeed, a universal coverage system that includes Medicare Advantage would no longer be a single-payer system. We'll return to this issue in Chapter 6, which deals explicitly with alternatives to M4A.

QUESTION #4: HOW DO DOCTORS AND HOSPITALS GET PAID?

As we hope has become clear throughout this book, if one wants to understand how the healthcare system works, follow the money. To a large extent, the flow of dollars determines the organization of our health system and influences what kind of care is delivered.

M4A legislation must answer two key questions about the flow of money. First, *how* are providers paid? And second, *how much* do they get paid?

What Payment Method to Use?

In terms of how M4A would pay providers, there are two basic options: M4A could build on Medicare's existing payment methods, or it could move to a system of "global budgets."

In the current Medicare program, doctors are generally paid a fee for each service they provide, based on a predetermined fee schedule set by Medicare. Hospitals are generally paid a fixed sum every time they admit a patient to the hospital, with the payment amount based on the patient's diagnosis. In addition to these traditional payment methods, Medicare has introduced a variety of "value-based" payment methods—for instance, accountable care organizations (ACOs) that try to reward health systems for reducing spending, "pay-for-performance" programs that give physicians a bonus if they meet certain quality metrics, or "bundled payment" programs that pay a lump sum for a full episode of care (e.g., a knee replacement plus rehab) rather than a separate fee for every part of the service.

Healthcare experts love to debate the merits or demerits of these different approaches. The early years of value-based payment reform often brought lofty expectations—for instance, a 2013 article in the *Washington Post* gushed that "ACOs may actually be the unicorns we've been waiting for, spreading their cost-saving magic throughout the health system."[20] But the evidence so far has been less dramatic: some value-based payment programs have trimmed costs by a few percentage points (e.g., bundled payments for surgeries, ACOs led by physicians), others have *increased* spending (e.g., ACOs led by hospitals), and some may even be harmful (e.g., certain pay-for-performance schemes).[21] Experts disagree on whether value-based payments still have untapped potential or are fundamentally misguided. Either way, some critics wrongly think that M4A would mean reverting to a pure fee-for-service payment system. In reality,

M4A could continue Medicare's ongoing efforts at payment reform, inheriting both its successes and its frustrations.

The second major option for M4A is to usher in a more fundamental change to our healthcare payment system by moving to a "global" form of payment. For instance, HR1384 would implement global operating budgets for hospitals: instead of paying hospitals for each admission, hospitals would be paid a lump sum to cover all operating expenses over a given period. In other words, we could pay hospitals like we pay fire departments: a global budget to fund all the services it provides to a community, rather than a separate check every time it puts out a fire.

Global hospital budgets would be a significant transformation from the existing payment system. First, hospitals would have almost no need for billing and coding staff. Instead of submitting untold thousands of claims to different insurance companies each week, hospitals would simply receive one lump sum payment. In other words, attention would be refocused on how to spend the money, rather than on building up armies of billers and coders to bring in the money. Second, while the fee-per-admission system encourages hospitals to stay full, global budgets encourage investments to keep patients healthy and out of the hospital. Third, global budgets make no distinction between profitable and unprofitable lines of business. In the status quo, services like psychiatry are often unprofitable for a hospital, which leads to a tilt toward more profitable specialties that bring in extra revenue. Under a global hospital budget, hospitals could plan and provide services according to the needs of its patient population, rather than according to which lines of business are profitable. Fourth, global budgets would give M4A a predictable and powerful method of managing cost growth. Finally, global budgets could make hospital finances more resilient. The COVID-19 pandemic revealed just how fragile our hospitals can be in the face of an economic shock: with the virus keeping the most lucrative patients at home, hospital revenue plummeted, and some even faced bankruptcy. Under a global budget, hospitals would have stable funding during a crisis, allowing them the flexibility to redeploy resources to meet public health needs without sacrificing revenue. And even in normal times, the stability of global budgets could help sustain rural hospitals that provide critical services to their communities but sometimes lack the patient volume to survive in a fee-for-service system.[22]

However, there are also risks to global budgets. Hospitals may try to decrease the care they provide to the sickest patients who require the most expensive care or might avoid expanding into communities with the greatest medical need. If hospitals are no longer rewarded for providing a higher volume of services, they might choose to perform fewer costly elective procedures, hampering patients' ability to access those services. Politically, global payment models also give more power to the health systems receiving the lump sum payments rather than to the front-line clinicians providing care, which may affect political support from clinicians.

A further question for global budget systems is how to fund capital investments, like building a new hospital wing. Under HR1384, hospitals could not use their global operating budget to fund capital investments; instead, there would be a separate funding process that awards grants for capital projects. Supporters of this provision argue that in the status quo, where capital investments are made disproportionately by the most profitable health systems, the result is that dominant systems simply become more dominant over time—and medical resources continue to concentrate in particular areas, contributing to health inequity. In contrast, proponents of a publicly controlled capital expenditure fund view it as a way to distribute capital resources according to population needs.

Finally, global hospital budgets are only one possible version of global payment. Alternatively, M4A could pay groups of providers a budget to cover *all* the healthcare costs for a defined population, including primary, specialty, and hospital care. A Massachusetts program using this style of population-based global payment has been able to slow cost growth, and Maryland is rolling out a similar program.[23] Details aside, the upshot is that by covering the entire population M4A would have tremendous ability to drive changes to the healthcare payment system, testing and scaling up models far more swiftly than is possible in our multi-payer environment.

How Much Should M4A Pay Providers?

Whether M4A builds on Medicare's current payment methods or moves to global budgets, a critically important decision is how much M4A should pay hospitals and doctors compared to the status quo.

Let's first consider a Medicare for All program based on Medicare's existing payment methods. In the status quo, Medicare payment rates are generally lower than private insurance rates, and Medicaid pays the lowest rates of all. (One exception is that Medicare and Medicaid pay similar hospital rates.) M4A would transition these disparate payments into one unified set of rates.

What's the right rate? This question has enormous political and economic implications, affecting the likelihood of support from doctors and hospitals as well as the overall costs of M4A.

Here's one proposal: at a minimum, M4A could use Medicare's current payment rates; at a maximum, M4A could use a weighted average of Medicare, Medicaid, and private insurance rates (the "all-payer average" rate).[24] The all-payer average rate is estimated to be approximately 107 percent of Medicare rates for physicians, and between 119 percent and 134 percent of Medicare rates for hospitals.[25] To take one example that fits within these bounds, during the 2020 presidential campaign Senator Elizabeth Warren outlined a plan to have M4A pay physicians at current Medicare rates and to pay hospitals at 110 percent of current Medicare rates.

How would hospitals and doctors be affected if they got paid for every patient a certain percentage of Medicare rates?

First, it's critical to remember that M4A would not simply change reimbursement rates and leave the rest of the healthcare system unchanged. Consider the simple equation we introduced previously: *Income = (Price × Quantity) – Operating Costs.* For many hospitals and doctors, M4A would decrease the average price received for each service. But M4A would also decrease operating costs by vastly streamlining administration and by reducing the costs of the prescription drugs that hospitals purchase. M4A would also increase the quantity of care that can be delivered by freeing up clinician time from administrative tasks and by expanding coverage—including bringing some 30 million more patients into the system by covering the uninsured. Hospitals are well equipped to serve these new patients: the average hospital occupancy rate is only 62 percent, and a mere 40 percent for rural hospitals.[26] Furthermore, under M4A hospitals and doctors would get paid for services they currently provide without compensation.

Second, there are likely to be wide variations in how different providers are affected by new M4A payment rates. Hospitals with monopoly power currently charge very high prices to privately insured patients, so they have more to lose from a move to M4A payment rates. More broadly, providers who see more privately insured patients have more to lose. In contrast, safety-net hospitals or primary care doctors who serve higher proportions of Medicaid or uninsured patients could even see overall reimbursements go up under M4A—after all, Medicaid physician payment rates are 30 percent lower on average than Medicare rates, and even lower in some states.[27] The impact on physicians would also vary widely by specialty. According to one estimate, dermatologists and radiologists could face a significant decline in overall reimbursements, while general medical doctors would likely see less of an impact.[28]

Furthermore, M4A payment rates could be adjusted to achieve desired policy outcomes. For instance, the fee schedule could be modified to implement a relative increase in payment to primary care providers. Similarly, moving to a fixed percentage of Medicare rates may hit specialist physicians the hardest—but if desired, it's also possible to pick rates such that specialists don't see as much of a pay cut. Rates could also be adjusted to incentivize providers to deliver services in communities with unmet medical need, particularly in rural and low-income urban areas.

If M4A adopted a global payment approach, the issues raised are somewhat different—instead of choosing reimbursement rates for different services, M4A would need to determine the size of the global budgets for different institutions or populations. One possibility would be to set global budgets at a level similar to current spending. The challenge with this approach is that it could implicitly continue unwarranted funding disparities across hospitals or populations, such as paying less to providers who treat Medicaid patients and more to hospitals that leverage market power to charge high prices. M4A could attempt to adjust for these disparities when setting initial budgets, or when determining how budgets should change over time.

QUESTION #5: HOW DOES M4A COVER PRESCRIPTION DRUGS?

Every major M4A proposal includes significant reforms to the way that Medicare pays for prescription drugs. The central goal is to allow Medicare to negotiate drug prices with pharmaceutical companies.

Allowing Medicare to negotiate drug prices is extraordinarily popular, with support from 86 percent of the public, including 80 percent of Republicans.[29] But negotiating drug prices is also more complicated than it sounds. The government can't simply ask drug companies for lower prices; Medicare needs a real source of leverage to bring drug companies to a deal.

One way to exert leverage is to say no: Medicare could simply decline to cover drugs that it deems too expensive. Some countries use this strategy; for instance, in the United Kingdom the National Institute for Health and Care Excellence (NICE) will cover only drugs deemed to deliver appropriate value in terms of the capacity to extend or improve life compared to the cost.

In the US context, it's likely that the "just say no" approach would lead to high-stakes political battles between Medicare and the pharmaceutical industry. Consider a hypothetical example: A pharmaceutical company releases a new cancer drug that extends life by an average of one year compared to the next-best treatment, and offers it to M4A at a price that is $300,000 more per patient. What if Medicare tries to negotiate a lower price but the pharmaceutical company refuses to capitulate? If Medicare just accepted the higher price we would be right back to the status quo. Alternatively, Medicare could refuse to cover the drug until the price is lowered, but then a high-stakes political standoff would likely ensue. There might be significant public pressure on the pharmaceutical company to lower the price—but with billions of dollars on the line and investors watching closely, the company might conclude that if they hold out long enough, Medicare will eventually capitulate. And they might be right: it's hard to imagine patients with cancer and their families being okay with their elected officials blocking access to important medication in the name of decreasing national health expenditures. Medicare is ultimately accountable to voters; pharma companies are ultimately accountable to shareholders. It's easy to imagine many cases where Medicare would capitulate first. On a more fundamental level, the "just say no" strategy puts patients in the middle of pricing negotiations, and some may be left without access to medications that they would benefit from.

Medicare has other options to exert leverage in pricing negotiations. Medicare could threaten to impose a tax on corporate sales or profits of companies that refuse to negotiate. (In 2019, the House of Representatives passed a drug price negotiation bill that included such a tax penalty, though the

Senate did not take it up.) HR1384 includes another aggressive option: if the pharma company refuses to negotiate, the government can grant a different company a license to produce the medication as a generic. This so-called competitive licensing provision essentially threatens a company's patent in order to compel price concessions.

These are powerful tactics that government under Medicare for All would need to exercise judiciously. One big question is how to determine when a price is reasonable and when it's time to deploy pressure on the drug company to bring the price down.

One method for determining a reasonable price is to look at the prices charged in other high-income nations, like Canada or countries in western Europe. A second method might be to determine a value-based price for the drug. This would mean assessing how much health benefit the drug provides, and then setting a price based on that benefit. Independent from M4A, there is a movement in health policy to shift toward this kind of value-based pricing for pharmaceuticals. For instance, the Institute for Clinical and Economic Review (ICER) is an independent research organization that evaluates the clinical effectiveness of drugs and proposes benchmark prices that reflect the underlying value to patients.[30] ICER benchmarks have been used in the private sector as the basis for drug price negotiations: for example, in May 2018 Sanofi/Regeneron agreed to lower the price for an injectable cholesterol medication to match its value-based benchmark.[31] M4A could apply a similar paradigm nationally, or it could adopt a different public process that helps assess the value of new drugs.

In sum, threats like tax penalties or competitive licensing could bring pharma companies to the negotiating table, and having criteria like a value-based price could provide predictability and guidance to the negotiating process.

But in any discussion of drug pricing there's an elephant in the room: if drugs are cheaper, would pharma companies have less incentive to make them?

You've probably heard the argument before. It takes a lot of money to do the research and development (R&D) needed to discover a new drug, and the risk of failure is high. Investors put money into pharmaceutical R&D because they know new drugs can be sold at a high price, which means high profits. If prices go down, there's less opportunity to turn a profit. The argument is that private investors will therefore put less money into R&D, and fewer drugs will be discovered.

This concern should be taken seriously. Biomedical advances can lead to enormous gains in health and longevity, and a well-functioning healthcare ecosystem should produce new and better treatments decade after decade. With this in mind, there are several considerations for M4A.

First, high prices don't always incentivize the production of new, innovative drugs. That's because we're often charged high prices for drugs that are *not* new or innovative. Consider the most lucrative drug in the world: Humira, an anti-inflammatory medication produced by AbbVie that's used to treat conditions like rheumatoid arthritis and inflammatory bowel disease. Humira was approved in 2002, with its patent set to expire in 2016. But instead of letting Humira's patent expire, AbbVie filed for *more* patents on all aspects of the drug, even though it was the very same medication approved in 2002! At the dawn of 2021, Humira is not just on patent—it's protected by *more than 100 patents*, some of which won't expire until 2034.[32] AbbVie has allegedly taken advantage of this prolonged monopoly to double the price of Humira from about $19,000 per patient per year in 2012 to $38,000 in 2018, a year where global sales of Humira reached $20 billion.[33] Moreover, when the makers of competing drugs started gearing up for a colossal legal fight to challenge these patents, AbbVie allegedly paid settlements to eight different companies in exchange for agreements to delay bringing competing products to market.[34]

The strategies used to defend Humira are all common tactics that drug companies use to exploit our patent system: "evergreening" to extend monopolies as long as possible, "patent thickets" to build a legal fortress around a drug, and "pay-for-delay" deals to fend off generic competitors. The result? High drug prices. Here's the critical point: these high prices *do not* incentivize the production of new, innovative drugs. They incentivize the deployment of innovative legal strategies that keep prices high without delivering important new benefits to patients. M4A could bring down these prices without significant harm to innovation.

Furthermore, even new drugs do not always bring meaningful therapeutic benefits. The goal of pharmaceutical R&D should be improving health, not simply maximizing the number of drugs brought to market. But our current pricing system has a mixed record on this score. For instance, pharma companies are often incentivized to produce "me-too" drugs—medications similar to existing medicines, which provide little to no additional therapeutic benefit—as opposed to true breakthroughs. These drugs carry little risk of failure and take far less effort to develop but can still be patented because of small differences from existing drugs. According to one estimate, only 20 percent of the R&D budget allocated to clinical trials goes to drugs that the Food and Drug Administration categorizes as a "significant improvement" over existing drugs, with 80 percent going to drugs without significant additional benefit.[35]

If M4A brought down the price of drugs that offer little or no clinical benefit beyond what's already available, it's possible that fewer of these drugs would be produced. That trade-off might be worth it: the absence of those drugs would likely have little impact on patient health, but the savings from lower prices across the board could be substantial. More generally, if M4A uses its negotiating power to award high drug prices only to truly innovative drugs, it could help make R&D more efficient by targeting resources toward novel drugs with the potential to significantly improve health.

Still, for the subset of truly new and innovative drugs, there remains a genuine risk that significantly lower prices could reduce private investment in beneficial R&D. In these cases, it's worth noting that the impact of lower drug prices on innovation under M4A would be blunted by the fact that M4A would also give patients significantly better access to these medications. This matters because the incentive to produce a drug depends on price *and* the number of prescriptions sold at that price *(Revenue = Price × Quantity)*. Medicare for All would significantly increase the quantity of prescriptions filled for the vast majority of drugs by improving Americans' ability to access medications—both by covering the uninsured and by reducing out-of-pocket costs for drugs.

Even so, if concerns about decreased private investment in innovative R&D are significant enough, M4A could use some of the savings from lower drug prices to fund increased public investment in R&D. Publicly funded research, performed in universities with the support of organizations like the National Institutes of Health, is what leads to much of our most important innovation. A recent analysis found that over the last twenty-five years, more than half of the most transformative drugs had their origins in publicly funded research.[36] Compared to privately funded research, publicly funded research is also more likely to produce first-in-class drugs.[37] In addition to boosting investment in basic research, public funding could be used to support the clinical trials that are needed to bring drugs to market; drugs that are created and developed using public funds could be immediately manufactured as low-cost generics.

This public funding may be particularly important for supporting the R&D of new medications of significant clinical value that may not be rewarded well on the market. Consider new antibiotics, for example. These medications are necessary to treat emerging antibiotic-resistant bacteria. However, because they are used for a short period, often only once per patient, there is less financial incentive to create them (by contrast, patients might inject Humira twice a month for years or longer). Furthermore, part of the value of new antibiotics comes from *not* using them unless absolutely necessary, which helps avoid resistance. These missing incentives for private investment are, in part, why experts argue we are woefully behind in the race against antibiotic-resistant bacteria.[38]

These R&D reforms could be enacted independently of M4A, but the justification for greater investment in public R&D is even stronger when M4A is responsible for negotiating prices and procuring drugs on behalf of the entire population.

QUESTION #6: HOW IS THE PROGRAM ADMINISTERED?

Many of the policy questions discussed in this chapter can be answered directly in the design of M4A legislation. But during the implementation of a Medicare for All program—and as healthcare continues to innovate and evolve in the coming decades—the program must be able to adapt. A key question for M4A is therefore how the program is administered and governed.

There are two key dimensions to this question. First, to what extent is M4A administered federally, and to what extent is it administered regionally or in the states? And second, how should we balance the political accountability of M4A against operational independence?

Federal, Regional, and State Roles

The current Medicare program is mostly administered at the federal level, but there are also regional Medicare offices with important roles. One option for administering M4A would be to build on this existing structure.

Alternatively, M4A could feature a greater role for states. The most decentralized option would be to administer M4A almost entirely through the states, with funding provided by the federal government to achieve M4A's aims. This option would give each state latitude in how to provide universal coverage to its residents—defining exactly which benefits are covered, how providers are paid, and what the role of private insurers will be. Though the federal government could restrict how M4A funds are used and require certain outcomes be met, it would allow for localized operational control. (This would be closer to what we might call Medicaid for All.) Indeed, state Medicaid programs have tremendously valuable experience, infrastructure, and local knowledge that could be leveraged toward the success of a M4A system. Creating a larger role for states might also have political benefits for legislators representing areas with more skepticism of the federal government.

A hybrid option is to have M4A's core health insurance benefits administered by the federal government but to give states other roles in administration—perhaps offering additional wrap-around benefits (either permanently or in response to local emergencies), or focusing on social services and case management. State Medicaid programs also perform some public health activities—for instance, the Michigan Medicaid program responded to the Flint water crisis by obtaining funding to remove lead from the homes of Medicaid patients.[39] Under M4A, these functions could remain with state Medicaid offices or could be folded into state and local public health departments. In general, a reasonable goal is to ensure that any important benefit or service provided by Medicaid today should either be provided by M4A, transferred to another state or local agency, or kept as part of a reformed Medicaid program.

Accountability vs. Independence

Another challenge is how to balance the political accountability of M4A against its operational efficiency and independence. On one end of the spectrum you could imagine Congress micromanaging the M4A program, making decisions about whether fees for outpatient cardiology visits should increase by 1 percent or 1.5 percent next year, or whether a new imaging technique should become a covered benefit. On the other end of the spectrum you could imagine appointing a completely independent federal agency to make all these decisions. Many plausible models fall somewhere in the middle.

A model with relatively more political accountability is the existing Medicare program, which is administered by the Centers for Medicare and Medicaid Services (CMS), an agency within the Department of Health and Human Services (HHS). The CMS administrator is appointed by the president and confirmed by the Senate, serving until she or he resigns or is replaced by the same or a new president. The Medicare program does maintain an independent advisory board—the Medicare Payment Advisory Commission, or MedPAC—but its role is to advise Congress on Medicare, and it does not hold independent decision-making authority. One option under M4A would be to increase the authority of MedPAC, which has earned trust within the federal government over its more than twenty years of operation.

Models for greater independence could also take after the Federal Reserve Board or the Federal Trade Commission. The Federal Reserve Board consists of seven members, appointed by the president and confirmed by the Senate, who serve staggered fourteen-year terms. The Fed functions mostly independently and has authority to set United States monetary policy. Another model is the Federal Trade Commission (FTC), headed by five commissioners nominated by the president and confirmed by the Senate, each serving a seven-year term. No more than three commissioners can be of the same political party. The FTC also has significant authority to make independent decisions. Under M4A, an analogous body could be given some authority in making decisions about what new services should be covered and where reimbursement levels should be set. However, each option comes with some obvious political challenges: for instance, the Affordable Care Act attempted to create an Independent Payment Advisory Board to play some of these roles, but it was so controversial it never got off the ground.

Beyond these structural considerations, part of M4A's administrative success will depend on sheer operational competence. The botched rollout of HealthCare.gov during implementation of the Affordable Care Act provides a cautionary tale, especially given that M4A is partly premised on restoring popular trust in the ability of government to set ambitious goals and achieve them. Medicare itself may provide a lesson here. The original Medicare program went into effect July 1, 1966; government leaders spoke of this date as "M-Day" and organized a highly successful effort to get the program up and running within eleven months of the legislation being signed. If M4A is passed into law, the political and human stakes of executing the implementation smoothly will be extraordinary.

QUESTION #7: HOW WILL WE TRANSITION TO MEDICARE FOR ALL?

Medicare for All would bring tens of millions of uninsured Americans fully into the healthcare system and would make it more affordable for so many more. To meet the task of providing care to the full population, M4A will need to quickly ramp up the clinical workforce. Given the existing primary care shortage, it will be especially important for M4A to bolster the primary care workforce. Many policy tools are available to do so: increasing the number of residency training slots, rebalancing payment rates for primary care versus specialty care, expanding loan forgiveness for primary care trainees, making it easier for physicians who immigrate to the United States to practice here, boosting training opportunities for nurse practitioners and physician' assistants, and more.

Though M4A will almost certainly mean more clinical jobs, it will also likely mean far fewer administrative jobs. Indeed, most private insurers will downsize or close, leaving many people without job prospects in the industry; this will similarly affect the armies of billers and coders in hospital and physician back offices. Many new administrative jobs are likely to be available with Medicare or its administrative contractors, but there will be significantly fewer administrative jobs than under the current system (indeed, reducing the need for administrative work is one way M4A reduces healthcare costs). A critical piece of the transition must include assistance for these workers; both HR1384 and S1129 set aside funds for this purpose. Job retraining and assistance with job placement will be important parts of this transition.

A further question is how many years it will take to transition from the current healthcare system to Medicare for

All. HR1384 proposes to make the transition over two years, while S1129 proposes a four-year transition. The question of how long to set aside for the transition is both practical and political. Practically, it will take time to get the program up and running, to finalize pertinent rules and regulations, and for providers to adjust to a new payment scheme. Politically, the risk of a short transition is that a botched rollout could hamper faith in the program—but a long transition could leave the program under attack if political winds change before it is fully built.

What needs to happen during the transition? Most obviously, people need to transition onto M4A coverage. One approach is to create a Medicare for All option that anyone can opt into during the transition period. The transition could also adopt principles of triage to provide assistance quickly to the uninsured. For instance, everyone under a certain income threshold could immediately be granted free access to the Medicare for All option, including the millions of Americans who live in states that have failed to expand Medicaid. Another transitional approach is to phase in Medicare for All by age—for instance, make all children and those over fifty-five eligible in the first year, and then expand coverage by ten-year age increments every year.

Other elements of reform can also be rolled out more quickly. New investments in the medical workforce could be made immediately, knowing that it takes many years to train each new clinician. New antitrust measures could be enforced immediately as well. The prescription drug negotiation system could be implemented as quickly as possible. Prices that hospitals are allowed to charge to private insurers might be capped to begin the transition to a new system of unified payment rates.

Medicare for All promises to provide comprehensive health insurance to all Americans under a single, publicly funded plan. To make that vision a reality, legislators and the public will need to confront a number of important policy questions with huge economic and political ramifications. If Medicare for All becomes law, the choices outlined in this chapter—what's covered, who's covered, how the system is organized—will reverberate for decades to come.

5

HOW TO PAY FOR IT

Every dollar spent on medical care is a dollar that comes out of someone's income, taken from a worker or a business owner or a shareholder or a family. So it's not quite right to say that "insurance companies" or "the government" pays our healthcare bills. *We* pay the premiums or the taxes—and usually both. Insurance companies and the government are the intermediaries that collect the money and send it where it needs to go. But the money comes from us, no matter the healthcare system. The American people fund our healthcare system today, and the American people would fund our healthcare system under Medicare for All. What changes under Medicare for All is the size of the national healthcare bill, where we send the money, who keeps some of it for profit (and how much they keep), and which people pay how much.

That last question—who pays how much—is also a question of social values. How much should the rich pay for healthcare compared to the middle class and the poor? How much should the healthy pay compared to the sick? Our current healthcare system takes an implicit stand on these questions, but the answers often remain hidden beneath a fog of complexity. M4A brings these ethical issues out of the shadows, forcing us to decide collectively which values should be embedded into a system that consumes nearly a fifth of our economy and takes care of us at our most fragile moments.

TODAY'S HEALTHCARE BILL

Under the current system, Americans are projected to share a $52 trillion healthcare bill during the 2020s, with annual expenditures above $4 trillion at the start of the decade and over $6 trillion by its close. We each contribute to that bill in three main ways: taxes, insurance premiums, and out-of-pocket costs. (Employees technically have a large chunk of their premiums covered by employers, but at the end of the day those premium payments come out of money set aside for employee remuneration. For instance, if your work is worth $75,000 a year to your employer, who has to chip in $15,000 for your insurance premium, your salary will only be $60,000.)

Most of these costs are hidden. We usually think of our healthcare costs as what we pay personally for premiums plus what we spend out of pocket during the year. But according to a study by the RAND Corporation, those costs make up just *one-fifth* of what we're really paying for healthcare.[1] Employer-paid premiums and healthcare taxes make up a far larger share of spending.

Indeed, employer-paid premiums function like a hidden tax, taking more and more money out of American paychecks every year. As a result, the hidden costs of healthcare are particularly stark for Americans with insurance through their jobs. If you have employer-based coverage and want to know how much you're really contributing to our multitrillion-dollar healthcare bill, here's one way to get an average estimate: take what you personally contribute to premiums and out-of-pocket costs, then *multiply by seven.*[2]

Americans spend a lot of money on insurance premiums and out-of-pocket costs. But we pay *far* more for healthcare through taxes and lost wages. These high costs are not distributed equitably. When all the taxes, premiums, and out-of-pocket costs are tallied, poor and middle-class Americans currently pay a *larger share* of their income for healthcare compared to the wealthy.[3] Every group in the bottom 60 percent of the income distribution is paying a larger share than any group in the top 40 percent. The top 1 percent are contributing a smaller share of their income than the bottom 20 percent.[4] On average, the poorest fifth of households are paying *more than a third of their income for healthcare.*[5]

Public healthcare programs like Medicare and Medicaid are financed at least somewhat progressively, with the top 10 percent of earners contributing a larger share of their income to these programs than the rest of the population. (Remember, *progressive* financing means richer people contribute a higher proportion of their income, like the federal income tax; *regressive* financing means poorer people contribute more as a proportion of income, like the sales tax.) That's because public programs are mostly financed by taxes, some of which are progressive.

In contrast, private healthcare spending is steeply regressive. Low-income Americans—those with a mean pretax compensation of roughly $40,000—contribute three times more of their total compensation to private healthcare costs compared to the highest earners.[6] Private healthcare spending is regressive because insurance premiums and out-of-pocket costs are regressive: a $20,000 insurance premium and a $5,000 deductible aren't much of a burden for a millionaire executive but might be a huge drag on the finances of a teacher or a nurse. The tax break for employer-based coverage makes our system even more regressive, giving a bigger windfall to people in the highest tax brackets.

Our current system also places a far larger financial burden on people who need more medical care. Americans in poor health have out-of-pocket costs three times higher than those in excellent health.[7] Some Americans might pay no out-of-pocket costs in a given year, while those with acute or chronic illness might spend many thousands of dollars.

High deductibles in particular have the effect of shifting costs onto people with the greatest medical needs. Many patients with chronic illnesses reliably spend up to their deductible year after year: for instance, they might need to take a high-cost medication over the course of many years, or they might have a condition like cystic fibrosis or sickle cell anemia that requires frequent hospital admissions. Because these patients predictably spend their entire deductible, high deductibles function like a tax on chronic illness.

This situation is ironic given the broad consensus that American health policy should provide strong protections for people with preexisting conditions. One of these protections is that insurance companies shouldn't be able to charge higher premiums to a person who has a preexisting condition. But high deductibles serve nearly the same role: people with preexisting conditions are likely to pay thousands of dollars more each year working their way through a high deductible.

MEDICARE FOR ALL

How would the costs of Medicare for All compare to the current system?

To answer this question, the first task is to determine what the total national healthcare bill would be under Medicare for All. This requires tallying up all the new costs of Medicare for All, including covering the uninsured, reducing out-of-pocket costs, and adding new benefits, and then subtracting the savings from reduced administrative costs and lower prices for drugs and medical services.

Between 2016 and 2020, at least ten different experts undertook detailed cost estimates of Medicare for All. Different analysts came to different conclusions: many experts found that national health spending under Medicare for All would be trillions of dollars *lower* over a decade than under the current system, while others estimated that Medicare for All would *increase* spending by trillions of dollars. Furthermore, the disparate cost estimates do not seem to simply reflect partisan bias. Charles Blahous, who formerly worked in George W. Bush's presidential administration, conducted a cost estimate for the Mercatus Center, a libertarian think tank that receives funding from the Koch brothers. The report found that Medicare for All would *decrease* national health spending by $2 trillion over ten years.[8] In contrast, the Urban Institute—a more liberal think tank—estimated that M4A would *increase* national health spending by $7 trillion over a decade.[9]

What explains these different conclusions? We saw one major reason in Chapter 4: there are different ways to design Medicare for All. When different experts estimated the costs of Medicare for All, they actually modeled different versions of the policy—the most important differences being in how much hospitals and doctors would be paid, how aggressively drug prices would be negotiated, and what benefits would be covered (in particular, whether or not long-term care is covered makes an enormous difference in the overall costs). Beyond these policy differences, analysts also made different assumptions about administrative savings; for instance, some assumed that M4A would cause Medicare's administrative costs to *increase* nearly threefold as a percentage of its budget (an assumption we find implausible), while others assumed

M4A's administrative costs would be 3 percent or less, similar to Medicare today.

Finally, analysts made different predictions about how much more healthcare people would use after gaining insurance or having their out-of-pocket costs reduced. We know that people use more healthcare when it costs them less, but economically it's difficult to predict exactly how large the nationwide effect would be under M4A. Because healthcare use is constrained by the supply of doctors and hospitals, the impact of M4A will also depend on how many new doctors enter the workforce, whether hospitals expand, and whether new facilities are built that wouldn't have otherwise existed.

Out of a $52 trillion pie, any detail that alters total spending by just 2 percent counts for $1 trillion per decade. There are many such details when it comes to Medicare for All—hence the range of estimates.

Even with this variation, virtually all these estimates fall within the same general range: in the decade after enactment, national health spending under Medicare for All would be similar to current health spending, *plus or minus 15 percent.*[10] To be sure, the dollar amount at stake in "plus or minus 15 percent" is enormous. It's also important to avoid false equivalence between competing estimates; for instance, it's likely that estimates at the high end of this range did not adequately account for administrative savings. More important is that these different estimates don't just reflect different economic guesses but depend critically on what's actually written into M4A legislation.

These recent cost estimates of M4A also build on a longer history of single-payer modeling. One comprehensive report examined twenty-two cost analyses conducted over thirty years estimating the cost of single-payer proposals at the state and federal levels, finding that nineteen of the estimates projected overall savings in the first year and that all suggested the potential for long-term cost savings.[11]

This evidence helps cut through some of the partisan rhetoric on single-payer healthcare. On one side, critics sometimes speak as if Medicare for All would launch our spending into the stratosphere. On the other side, supporters sometimes hope that because single-payer systems in other countries are half as expensive as our current system, Medicare for All would swiftly cut our health spending in half. Neither of these scenarios is likely. The evidence paints a less dramatic picture: national health spending under Medicare for All could be somewhat higher or somewhat lower than under current law, depending on how the program is designed. But it is possible to cover all Americans under Medicare for All without spending more than we do now, if that's a goal that legislators and the public seek to achieve.

Furthermore, it's likely that Medicare for All would decrease the yearly growth rate of healthcare costs—and therefore reduce healthcare costs over the long term. That's because Medicare for All has more tools to contain spending over time, like putting more control on how quickly hospital payment rates and drug prices go up. For instance, per-person spending in Medicare increased just 20 percent from 2008 to 2018, while per-person spending in private insurance increased by 50 percent.[12] Furthermore, since 2000, payment rates for hospital care and emergency department visits have grown far more rapidly in private insurance than in Medicare.[13] For this reason, ten-year projections are likely to underestimate the savings of Medicare for All. Over the long term, Medicare for All presents a powerful opportunity to finally get a hold on runaway spending growth.

To illustrate how all these forces come together, consider the Medicare for All proposal released by Senator Elizabeth Warren's 2020 presidential campaign. On the benefits side, Warren's plan adopted the comprehensive benefits of Bernie Sanders's S1129 bill, including long-term care, dental, vision, and hearing, and virtually no out-of-pocket costs. To rein in prices, Warren proposed paying physicians at existing Medicare rates and paying hospitals at Medicare rates plus 10 percent. She also proposed steep cuts to drug prices, as much as 70 percent for brand-name drugs. The experts who evaluated the plan for Warren's campaign estimated that the generous expansion of coverage and the aggressive cost control measures nearly cancelled each other out: national health spending under her Medicare for All plan was projected to be just below the $52 trillion per decade projected under current law.[14]

How much would this kind of Medicare for All plan "cost"? From the perspective of the American public as a whole, the additional cost of Warren's version of M4A would be zero dollars. (Or less.) Every dollar of healthcare spending is a dollar that comes from someone's income: the American public could pay $52 trillion during the 2020s for our current healthcare system, or they could pay $52 trillion for M4A. The total cost is $52 trillion; the additional cost is zero. If anything, the cost to the American public is negative.

What changes is the path those dollars take to get from the bank accounts of the public into the hands of hospitals, doctors, and drug companies—and what these dollars buy. Under Medicare for All, the vast majority of that $52 trillion would be channeled through the federal government before being sent to its final destination in the healthcare system.

So when the *New York Times* ran the headline "Elizabeth Warren Proposes $20.5 Trillion Health Care Plan," one translation is that $20.5 trillion in healthcare spending would be channeled through the government instead of through private insurers.[15] (The $20.5 trillion in additional federal spending is less than the $52 trillion total mostly because the government already finances more than half of the nation's healthcare spending, and also because some types of healthcare spending—like over-the-counter medical supplies and state spending on public health—would not be absorbed by Medicare for All.)

It's notable that less of that $52 trillion would find its way into the marketing departments of large corporations, the salaries of insurance company CEOs, the administrative budgets of insurers and providers, or the bank accounts of insurance company shareholders—places where nearly a quarter of our dollars end up today.[16] Instead, a larger proportion would go into caring for patients, including the roughly 30 million Americans without insurance coverage under the current system who would be covered under Medicare for All.

This shift toward patient care is reflected in the ledger of the costs and savings under Medicare for All. One of the largest sources of savings under M4A is administrative efficiency: streamlining insurance overhead, and also reducing the administrative costs of providers. In contrast, virtually all the new costs under M4A represent new spending on clinical care: covering the Americans who are uninsured, making care more affordable for those with insurance, and covering new benefits like vision, dental, and long-term care. If national health spending stays about the same under M4A but we spend trillions less on administration, that means *more* total dollars will be spent on medical services: hospital care, physician services, nursing facilities, home healthcare, prescription drugs, and more. M4A does not starve the healthcare system of funds; instead, it redirects more of what we're spending already into actual care.

PAYING FOR IT

Even if M4A costs the American public about the same as the current system, how we pay for healthcare—and who pays how much—would change substantially. Trillions of dollars would be shifted from insurance company balance sheets onto the government budget. How would the government raise the necessary funds?

Financing the Status Quo

First, let's look at how we pay for healthcare right now. There are four main streams of healthcare financing in the status quo: the federal government, state and local governments, employers, and families. Although all the money ultimately comes from individuals, that money flows through these four streams.

Many Americans would be surprised to learn that the government *already* finances the majority of healthcare spending in the United States: in 2017, public sources financed 61 percent of healthcare spending, and private spending financed 39 percent.[17] (That's a big reason healthcare costs are hidden today: we already pay for most of the healthcare system through taxes.) The federal government financed 44 percent of the nation's healthcare spending. Much of this spending goes toward Medicare, Medicaid, and nearly a dozen other public programs. But the federal government also spends a considerable sum of money subsidizing private health insurance, including subsidies on the ACA marketplace and the tax break for employer-based insurance. Indeed, in 2017 the federal government spent nearly $280 billion subsidizing employer insurance—the largest expenditure in the entire tax code, worth about $1,800 for each person with job-based coverage.[18] State and local governments financed another

17 percent of national health spending. Perhaps surprisingly, state and local governments spend almost as much on private insurance premiums for government employees as they do on Medicaid. All told, according to one estimate nearly 98 percent of Americans with health coverage have their insurance paid for or subsidized by taxpayers.[19]

Private sector spending is split between employers and families. Employers contribute to the insurance premiums of their employees; families pay insurance premiums as well as out-of-pocket costs when they receive care. The financing of private health insurance is steeply regressive. For instance, lower-income families with job-based coverage spend *three times* as much as a proportion of income on premiums and out-of-pocket costs compared to higher-income families: families below 200 percent of the poverty line spend 14 percent of their income on these costs, while those above 400 percent of the poverty line spend just 4.5 percent.[20]

Financing Medicare for All

M4A would significantly change the way that the burden of healthcare costs is spread across the population. The details of M4A financing proposals are likely to evolve as they move through legislative and political debate. But there are two basic elements likely to serve as the foundation to any M4A financing plan: repurposing existing public funds, and replacing private healthcare spending with progressive taxes.

Repurposing Existing Government Funds

The primary way to pay for M4A is to use money the government is already spending on healthcare. The federal government already finances almost half the nation's healthcare spending. M4A can combine existing federal spending on Medicare, Medicaid, and private insurance subsidies into a single stream to be used for M4A.

One choice that will need to be made is whether states should contribute the money they currently spend on Medicaid programs and private insurance premiums into the overall M4A pool. Capturing this money would decrease the amount of new revenue that needs to be raised at the federal level. On the other hand, leaving this money with the states would allow them to direct the funds to other programs that have been crowded out by Medicaid over the past several decades, such as public education. Alternatively, if M4A was administered at the state level (an option described in Chapter 4), this money could be left with the states and also repurposed to cover M4A.

In any case, *existing* government funds would provide the single largest source of financing for M4A.

Replacing Private Healthcare Spending with Progressive Taxes

Combined with existing public funds, the second major way to pay for M4A is to replace existing private healthcare spending with progressive taxes. There are three general ways to raise this money: capture some or all of the money that employers currently spend on healthcare, capture some or all of the money that families currently spend on healthcare, or raise revenue from new sources.

Today, employers might send a portion of payroll each month to Aetna or Blue Cross to fund insurance premiums for workers. Under a Medicare for All payroll tax, employers would continue to send a portion of payroll each month to fund insurance for workers—but the check would be sent to Medicare. In that way, a payroll tax levied on employers would replicate the way that employer-based premiums are currently paid for.

A reasonable policy goal is to ensure that in total, *less* money comes out of payroll to fund health insurance under M4A than in the status quo. Even so, the shift from our current system to a payroll tax would create winners and losers. Businesses with higher-income employees have an advantage in the current system, because healthcare costs represent a smaller fraction of payroll. Replacing regressive insurance premiums with a flat or progressive payroll tax would likely benefit businesses with low-income employees; those with high-income employees might end up worse off (depending, of course, on the level of the tax).

Family spending on premiums and out-of-pocket costs could be replaced by an income tax, a payroll tax, a Medicare for All premium (standardized or income-based to make it progressive), or a value-added tax. (Common in European countries, a value-added tax is similar to a sales tax but is levied at each stage of production, rather than just at the point of final sale.) Instead of regressive premiums and out-of-pocket costs, most of these options could be designed to be progressive, thereby saving money for the middle class and the poor.

A reasonable policy goal would be to have any new taxes on middle-class or low-income families be lower than what these families currently pay for healthcare. One challenge for this approach is the considerable variability in what families currently pay for care—in particular, people with greater medical needs might pay thousands of dollars in annual out-of-pocket costs, while other Americans pay zero out-of-pocket costs in a given year. For this reason, any such taxes could be designed to be less than what most families spend on premiums alone, not taking into account out-of-pocket costs.

M4A could also be financed through new progressive taxes that are not meant to replace existing healthcare spending but are designed to bring in money from new sources. Proposals in this category include a wealth tax on the richest Americans, raising the marginal income tax rate on the highest earners, reforming the corporate tax code, a financial transactions tax, taxing income from investments at the same rate as income from work, and a variety of other reforms to broaden the tax base. A full analysis of the strengths and weaknesses of these various proposals is beyond our scope here. But the key point is that there are multiple options for M4A financing that don't place a large burden on the middle class or the poor.

Putting It All Together

What would a financing plan with these elements look like in practice?

Elizabeth Warren's 2020 presidential campaign released one of the most detailed Medicare for All financing plans to date, which we can consider as an illustrative example. As described previously, national health spending under the Warren version of M4A is projected to be $52 trillion throughout the 2020s (an amount that is just under the status quo). Most of this spending would be financed using existing public sources: most existing federal healthcare spending would be shifted to Medicare for All, and states would be required to contribute to Medicare for All an amount similar to what they would spend under current law on Medicaid and private insurance for government employees. That leaves $20.5 trillion in new federal spending required over ten years. Employers would supply $9 trillion through an "employer Medicare contribution" equivalent to 98 percent of what they currently spend on health insurance premiums. The remaining $11 trillion would be raised with a variety of taxes levied on large corporations and the wealthiest households, including a tax on wealth over $1 billion. Critically, these new taxes on corporations and the wealthy would replace the $11 trillion that families are currently projected to spend on insurance premiums and out-of-pocket costs in the status quo; under Warren's financing plan, families would keep that $11 trillion.

In essence, employers would spend about the same under the Warren Medicare for All plan as they would spend in the status quo, and federal and state governments would shift their current healthcare spending into M4A. But nearly $11 trillion in healthcare costs would be shifted from American families onto large corporations and the wealthy.

Senator Bernie Sanders's 2020 presidential campaign published a set of financing options that shed light on Sanders's general philosophy of how single-payer healthcare could be financed. Employer spending on private insurance could be replaced by a 7.5 percent income-based premium (essentially a payroll tax) levied on employers. To protect small businesses, the first $1 million of payroll would be exempted. Employee healthcare spending could be replaced by a 4 percent income-based premium paid by individuals. To protect low-income workers, the first $29,000 of income would be exempted from this requirement. Additional revenue could be raised through a variety of progressive taxes aimed at the wealthy: making the income tax and the estate tax more progressive, taxing capital gains at the same rate as ordinary income, limiting tax deductions for the wealthy, instituting a wealth tax, and/or reforming the corporate tax system. The Sanders campaign estimated that these revenue sources would provide approximately $17.5 trillion over ten years.[21]

THE KITCHEN TABLE BUDGET

For most Americans, what really matters is the "kitchen table" budget: how much does your family spend on healthcare each month, and how much is left over for other priorities? A focus on the kitchen table budget—rather than the government budget or overall national health spending—highlights how M4A would impact the finances of individuals and families.

The impact of Warren's version of M4A on kitchen table budgets is straightforward: families would save what they currently spend on premiums and out-of-pocket costs. Since these costs are projected to total $11 trillion over the 2020s, Warren's presidential campaign said her plan "would mark one of the greatest federal expansions of middle class wealth in our history."[22]

Some of Warren's taxes on the wealthy could impact middle-class finances indirectly—for instance, higher taxes on businesses might be partly passed on to workers over the long term. But for the middle class, these indirect effects are overwhelmed by the direct savings from eliminating $11 trillion in healthcare costs.

The Sanders approach to financing M4A bears many similarities in terms of the kitchen table budget. Families would save on insurance premiums and out-of-pocket costs; in exchange, they would pay a 4 percent income-based premium for M4A. Because private insurance is financed regressively, this change is likely to produce savings for middle-class and low-income families, while high-income families would likely pay the same or more for M4A than they do today. Employer spending on insurance premiums would be replaced by an income-based premium that functions as a flat payroll tax—again, middle-class and low-income workers (and their employers) are likely to benefit from this change, while high-income workers (and their employers) would likely end up paying more.

The detailed effects of this general financing approach are demonstrated by a report from the nonpartisan RAND Corporation, which performed a detailed economic study of a single-payer plan for New York State.[23] The New York single-payer plan would be financed through progressive payroll taxes as well as non-payroll taxes. The researchers found that overall healthcare costs would decline slightly under the single-payer plan, perhaps just 1 percent savings in the short term. But the researchers found that on average, 90 percent of households—those making $291,000 a year or less—would save money under the single-payer plan. Households in the bottom 75 percent of income would save an average of $3,000 in healthcare costs; families below 139 percent of the federal poverty level would see their healthcare costs fall by half. These remarkable findings emphasize that healthcare affordability depends not just on systemwide costs but on how those costs are distributed—there is no plausible way to cut costs in half for low-income families without changing the underlying cost distribution.

The bottom line is that if your M4A taxes are lower than what you currently pay for healthcare, you'll save money under M4A. M4A could be designed to ensure that virtually all middle-class and low-income families come out ahead on average, raising taxes but reducing healthcare costs even more. Warren's financing plan also shows that it's not strictly necessary to raise middle-class taxes to finance M4A.

From an economic point of view, the Warren and Sanders approaches have different strengths and weaknesses, but the upshot is that there is a range of feasible options to fund M4A. The difference between their plans is as much about politics as economics. The Warren plan is specifically designed to avoid raising taxes on the middle class. In contrast, the pitch made by Sanders is that middle-class taxes will go up, but total healthcare costs will go down.

Many people fear that raising middle-class taxes is political kryptonite. Others see middle-class taxes as an indispensable tool to build long-term support for public programs. Perhaps both have elements of truth, where programs funded by the middle class are both more difficult to pass and more resilient once in place. Reflecting on his administration's Social Security program, Franklin D. Roosevelt explained: "We put those [payroll taxes] there so as to give the contributors a legal, moral, and political right to collect their pensions and their unemployment benefits. With those taxes in there, no damn politician can ever scrap my social security program. Those taxes aren't a matter of economics, they're straight politics."[24]

CONCLUSION

The airwaves are filled with competing claims about Medicare for All driving healthcare costs into the stratosphere or quickly slashing our costs to the international average. Neither of these outcomes is likely. Depending on how Medicare for All is designed—particularly how comprehensive the coverage is and how much the program reimburses for prescription drugs and medical care—total healthcare costs could be modestly lower or higher than costs in the status quo, at least over the medium term. Since a single payer has more tools than our current system to control cost growth over time, over the long term the savings from Medicare for All are likely to be more significant.

M4A would also have a tremendous impact on where our healthcare dollars are spent and how those costs are shared across the population. Our current system funnels a sizable portion of healthcare dollars to pay the overhead costs of insurance companies and providers, and it places an outsized burden on Americans with lower incomes and greater medical need. M4A focuses more of these dollars on patient care, and it could make healthcare much more affordable for families who find themselves financially or medically insecure in our current system. Replacing high deductibles and regressive private insurance premiums with progressive taxes also reflects a broader effort under M4A to transform healthcare from a consumer product into a public good.

Healthcare consumes nearly a fifth of the American economy. The highly technical debate about how to pay for M4A masks a fundamental truth: behind the number crunching, Medicare for All expresses a new vision for economic justice.

6

MEDICARE FOR ALL VS. ALTERNATIVES

There's more than one path to universal coverage. But some of those paths would leave behind people like Lisa Cardillo. In her thirties with three children, Lisa had "good" private insurance but still suffered a raft of unaffordable medical bills and years of battling insurance companies after she survived a cardiac arrest. Reforms that focus exclusively on increasing the number of people with insurance would provide no relief to the 160 million Americans like Lisa who have private insurance through an employer. They also do nothing about the challenges faced by people who get their coverage from Medicaid, Medicare, or the Affordable Care Act marketplaces. To be sure, it is an enormous problem that tens of millions of Americans have no health insurance—but that's just one symptom of the larger structural problems we have detailed in this book.

In addition to lack of insurance, in Chapter 1 we outlined a fuller set of major problems that Americans face in our current system: our healthcare is too expensive, too many Americans can't access the care they need, we're sicker than we should be, and the experience of giving and receiving care is eroding. When analyzing how health reform proposals do (or do not) address these problems, it is also helpful to keep in mind the "active ingredients" of Medicare for All described in Chapter 3. To review the six key elements of M4A:

1. *Universal coverage.* M4A guarantees health coverage to every American.
2. *Comprehensive coverage.* M4A guarantees that Americans' health coverage is comprehensive in terms of the range of covered benefits, the availability of a wide range of clinicians and hospitals, and minimal or no financial barriers to receiving care.
3. *Pricing power.* M4A can wield its considerable negotiating leverage to rein in the cost of drugs, hospital stays, and physician services.
4. *Administrative efficiency.* M4A eliminates the high overhead costs of private insurance companies and reduces the administrative burden on providers and patients.
5. *Progressive financing.* M4A allows healthcare to be financed progressively, replacing the regressive financing of private insurance.

6. *Public accountability*. M4A would be accountable to the American public, rather than shareholders.

When evaluating alternative reforms, it's also helpful to distinguish three functions of a health insurer, whether private or public: funding the insurance pool, administering the insurance plan, and deciding how much to pay for services. Under private insurance, all three functions are generally private: private insurance premiums, private management, and privately negotiated payment rates. Under Medicare for All, all three functions would be public: tax financing, public management, and publicly determined payment rates. As we'll see, reform proposals that stop short of M4A often seek to mix and match public and private responsibility for these three insurer functions.

Of course, history and politics cast a shadow over any policy discussion of M4A relative to its alternatives. In particular, the failure of the Clinton reform in the 1990s led many strategists to treat incremental reform as politically necessary, as well as to favor plans that are acceptable to the healthcare industry in order to allay the all-out attacks that spoiled reform for much of the twentieth century. The Affordable Care Act is often viewed as a vindication of this political strategy, and these same suppositions color the debate about Medicare for All. As a result, health reform debates are inevitably influenced by both policy and political considerations—for instance, a greater role for private insurance could be justified by a genuine belief in the wisdom of organizing the healthcare system around private insurers, or based on a political judgment that it's not worth arousing the opposition of the private insurance industry. In Part III we examine these political considerations in detail, but in this chapter we focus on the policy substance of the alternatives to Medicare for All.

FIX UNINSURANCE: BUILD ON THE AFFORDABLE CARE ACT

The Affordable Care Act expanded health coverage in two main ways: expanding Medicaid to cover people with low incomes and creating marketplaces where people can buy private insurance using subsidies provided by the federal government. In terms of the three functions of insurers, the approach taken in the ACA marketplaces is to keep all insurance functions private but to regulate insurance companies more closely and to add on public subsidies to help people afford the private premiums. In the nonelderly population, the ACA pushed the insured rate from 82 percent in 2010 to a high of 90 percent in 2016.[1]

The uninsured rate could be reduced even further using a series of measures that build on the framework of the ACA: implement Medicaid expansion in all states, expand subsidies to buy private insurance on the ACA marketplaces, ensure that more people eligible for coverage actually get enrolled, and cover undocumented immigrants.[2]

This package of reforms to build on the ACA could move the United States close to universal coverage. Indeed, states like Massachusetts have taken many of these steps—expanding Medicaid, adding coverage options for undocumented immigrants—and in 2018 Massachusetts had one of the lowest uninsured rates in the nation, at approximately 3 percent.[3] In a fragmented insurance system it is difficult to truly end uninsurance—for instance, some people will lose Medicaid coverage when they get a raise, and others will lose their employer-based insurance if they leave their job, resulting in gaps where people have no coverage. Still, by building on the ACA we can get close to solving the problem of uninsurance.

But every other problem in US healthcare would remain untouched. Our healthcare would remain the most expensive in the world, with unaffordable prices and high administrative costs. Uninsurance would no longer be a barrier to care, but the march of high deductibles and other financial barriers would continue. Our healthcare financing system would continue to harm the poor and marginalized, and our fragmented system would continue to place a heavy burden on clinicians and patients.

Put differently, a reform plan that only builds on the ACA lacks nearly all the active ingredients of Medicare for All: although we could approach universal coverage, coverage would not become more comprehensive, the public would not gain negotiating leverage against the healthcare industry to rein in prices, administrative efficiency would not be improved, financing would remain regressive, and accountability to shareholders would be retained.

Finally, a system that builds on the ACA alone is likely to remain inequitable. The ACA marketplaces separate insurance plans into four "metal levels": platinum, gold, silver, and bronze. People who can afford platinum plans enjoy comprehensive health coverage, while people with bronze plans are saddled with deductibles so high they might not be able to afford care altogether. Any system that explicitly stratifies Americans into markedly different classes of coverage is more likely to exacerbate health inequities, rather than solve them.

MARKET-BASED REFORMS

Expensive healthcare is one of the most serious problems in our system. A different approach to health reform is to try to make healthcare work more like other markets, relying on the forces of competition and choice to keep prices and costs under control. Proponents of market-based reform often agree that American healthcare today is far from a well-functioning marketplace. But they posit that with the right reforms, market forces could work in healthcare like they do elsewhere in our economy.

There are many examples of market-based reform proposals. Let's look at proposals that seek to reduce costs in two areas: hospitals and prescription drugs.

Mergers have enabled hospitals to charge higher prices to privately insured patients. In response, one proposal is to use antitrust laws against hospitals more aggressively to reduce the number of mergers. Hospitals could also be prohibited from proposing insurance contracts that hamper competition. One specific reform would be to prohibit hospitals from using "all-or-nothing" contracts that cover all the different hospitals owned by the same parent company, and instead to require that each hospital negotiate with insurers individually; another reform would be to ban contracts that block insurers from steering their members to lower-priced hospitals. Regulators could also loosen the requirement that insurance plans maintain an "adequate network" of hospitals and doctors, which would make it easier for insurance companies to create narrow networks that exclude high-priced hospitals.

Compared to our current system, these reforms would likely reduce hospital prices at least modestly. But a major challenge is that 90 percent of hospital markets are *already* highly concentrated.[4] Efforts to slow hospital consolidation would likely have limited ability to bring down prices in areas where one or two health systems already dominate the market. In areas where a meaningful range of doctors and hospitals is available, reforms that make it easier for insurance companies to exclude providers from their covered network could give insurers more leverage to negotiate lower prices. However, in Chapter 1 we described how insurance companies don't always have the incentive to fight for lower hospital prices: for instance, their profits are limited by law to a certain percentage of overall revenue, so a system of high prices and high premiums works well for many insurers. This is especially true in markets dominated by one or two insurance companies. With few competitors, insurance companies are less worried about patients switching to a plan with lower prices and premiums. In cases where insurance companies are able to negotiate lower prices by leaving more providers out of their covered network, these narrow networks come with their own downsides: patients are left with restricted choices, the system becomes more complex to navigate, there is a greater risk of surprise out-of-network bills, and patients with less ability to pay for comprehensive insurance are left with more limited access to care.

But on a more fundamental level, greater competition between hospitals is not sufficient to make hospital care function like a normal market good. All the unique features of healthcare that prevent it from being a true market good, as detailed in Chapter 1, still apply: for instance, as patients we usually have limited information about the services we need, we are often forced to make decisions under time pressure or with our health on the line, insurance covers most of the bill, and we care about more than price when making crucial decisions about our own health or the health of a loved one. Hospitals can take advantage of all these features to charge high prices, even if there are several competing hospitals in the area. When Lisa Cardillo had a mechanical heart pump placed after she went into shock in the intensive care unit, for example, it didn't much matter if another nearby hospital charged a lower price for the same procedure.

Market-based reforms are also available to tackle prescription drug prices. In the current system, pharma companies that sell patented drugs use a variety of tactics to limit competition from generics, like "patent thickets" that block competition by erecting a complex legal fortress around a drug, or "pay-for-delay" deals where one drug company pays another to keep a generic competitor off the market. Legislators could crack down on these practices. Another market-based reform is to loosen requirements for what drugs must be covered by insurance plans, giving insurers more power to leave expensive medications off their lists of covered drugs.

Improving competition from generic drugs by cracking down on abuses of the patent system is a good idea that would lower prices for some medications, and these reforms should be pursued whether under M4A or under our current system. Giving insurers more power to exclude expensive drugs from their plans could have a modest effect on prices, but only at the cost of preventing patients from accessing medicines they could benefit from. On a more fundamental level, when it comes to prescription drugs the power of competition is inherently limited: at the end of the day, the vast majority of drug spending goes to products that are protected by patents, meaning that direct competition is prohibited by law.

Though this is not a comprehensive ledger of all possible market-based attempts to reduce healthcare prices, the theme is clear: changing the rules of the market would likely reduce the prices for some healthcare services at least modestly, with the trade-off that some patients could lose access to certain providers or medications—after all, marketplaces are deliberately designed to ration goods and services based on willingness and ability to pay, rather than medical need. Furthermore, limited competition between providers or drugmakers is only one reason healthcare doesn't function like a normal market product.

If it is true that much of healthcare cannot be made into a normal market good, that's a strong reason to look toward regulation instead of competition to control healthcare costs.

FIX HIGH PRICES: PRICE REGULATION

We've already explained how Medicare for All could use its leverage to bring down the price of hospital stays, doctor visits, and prescription drugs. But perhaps we could tackle high prices without moving to Medicare for All: the existing insurance system could remain in place, but the government could set the prices across the entire healthcare system, including the prices charged to privately insured patients. In terms of the three functions of insurers, this approach would maintain private funding and administration of health insurance but would introduce publicly determined payment rates.

A limited version of price regulation would be to cap the prices that hospitals are allowed to charge to privately insured patients. The most comprehensive version of price regulation would be to directly determine the prices paid for *all* services. This approach is known as *all-payer rate-setting,* because the government would set payment rates for all payers—private insurers as well as public programs like Medicare and Medicaid.

All-payer rate-setting shares many of the cost-control strengths as Medicare for All: government uses its power to counteract the monopoly power and market failures that lead to extraordinarily high prices in our current system. All-payer rate-setting could bring down the prices of hospital care and doctor visits. The government could also negotiate drug prices on behalf of all insurers.

Compared to Medicare for All, all-payer rate-setting would have a more limited ability to reduce prices without affecting clinical care. Remember our simple equation: *Income = (Price × Quantity) – Operating Costs.* A single-payer system would significantly reduce operating costs for hospitals and physician practices by simplifying administration; Medicare for All can capture these savings for the taxpayer through reduced reimbursement rates, without affecting the real incomes of providers. Under all-payer rate-setting, there would simply be less administrative savings to capture. Furthermore, providers could see more patients under Medicare for All because time spent on administrative tasks would decline and coverage would become universal and comprehensive. Increased revenue from higher volume (plus the elimination of uncompensated care) would help counteract losses from lower payment rates. All-payer rate-setting doesn't expand coverage, meaning that price reductions would have a larger impact on providers' bottom lines. The same dynamic applies to prescription drugs: it is easier to cut drug prices without affecting innovation when reform also makes drugs far more accessible in the population at large.

The state of Maryland has used a version of all-payer rate-setting, and its experience shows the limitations of regulating prices without changing the underlying structure of the health insurance system. Although Maryland is among the richest states in the country, 7 percent of its nonelderly adults remain uninsured, and care remains unaffordable for many.[5] Indeed, Johns Hopkins Hospital in Baltimore has sued thousands of patients for unpaid medical debt, including low-income patients, even garnishing their wages and bank accounts.[6] Among communities of color in Baltimore, 33 percent have medical debt in collections.[7] In a regressively financed system that leaves patients uninsured and underinsured, all-payer rate-setting is no panacea.

Like the market-based reforms discussed earlier, price regulation is focused on cost rather than coverage. These cost-focused reforms—whether based on markets or regulation—could be combined with the ACA reforms discussed previously to increase coverage. Taken together, these reforms could achieve near-universal coverage and could decrease some healthcare prices. And if medical and drug prices fall, the savings could be passed on through lower premiums and deductibles. Still, coverage may not become significantly more comprehensive than it is today, many healthcare prices would remain high (particularly under market-based approaches), costly administrative complexity would persist, the system would continue to be financed regressively, and health insurance would not be publicly accountable.

PUBLIC OPTION (FOR SOME)

A public option is an insurance plan created by the government that people can choose to purchase. The public option was originally proposed as part of the ACA, and by the late 2010s it was commonly framed as a moderate alternative to Medicare for All.

In its narrowest version, a public option could be made available only to people who currently buy their insurance on the individual ACA marketplaces. This public option could be offered either by the federal government (perhaps a version of Medicare) or by state governments (perhaps a version of Medicaid—a so-called Medicaid buy-in). This is essentially an incremental way to strengthen the ACA: its main effect would be to make insurance somewhat more affordable for the roughly 11 million individuals who purchase insurance on the ACA marketplaces.

It is important to recognize that this kind of public option would *not* achieve universal coverage. Indeed, the nonpartisan Congressional Budget Office has projected that this kind of narrow public option by itself would have no meaningful effect on the number of people with health insurance.[8] A few million would switch from private to public coverage, but the uninsured would remain uninsured. Despite this drawback, this kind of public option is often falsely promoted as a way to achieve universal coverage and guarantee healthcare as a right.

PUBLIC OPTION FOR ALL

A broader version of the public option would be a public insurance plan that can be purchased by anyone, including people who currently get health coverage through an employer. (If the public plan offered is a version of Medicare, this type of proposal is sometimes called a Medicare buy-in.) Like M4A, a public option could be designed in numerous ways, which means many of the questions outlined in Chapter 4 also apply: What benefits would be covered? How much would beneficiaries need to pay out of pocket for care? How would doctors and hospitals be paid? A further critical question is how much the premium would be for the public option and what sort of subsidies would be available. These details matter enormously. But even without these details, the public option can be compared in general terms to Medicare for All.

A public option or a Medicare buy-in would not guarantee universal coverage: after all, people would still need to buy in. Even with subsidies, many people could still find a public option to be too expensive. And retaining a complex system of coverage options would likely mean that many people would find themselves between insurance plans when circumstances change, or would simply not enroll in coverage even if they are eligible for subsidies—one of the major problems we face in our current system.

The public option has several of the same active ingredients as Medicare for All. A public option could make coverage more comprehensive if the plan is designed to have low out-of-pocket costs or if benefits are expanded beyond what most private insurance plans currently cover. A public option may also have more negotiating power than private insurers to rein in prices for doctors, hospitals, and prescription drugs—at least for people who are enrolled in the public option. A public option would not make significant progress in improving administrative efficiency: although the public option itself is likely to have low administrative costs, private insurers would persist with their high administrative spending, and providers would still incur the significant administrative burden of interacting with a multitude of insurers. Financing could become somewhat more progressive depending on the nature of the subsidies for the public option, but regressive out-of-pocket costs might continue to play a large role and the regressive financing structure of employer-based insurance would remain in place. Public accountability would increase somewhat, but private insurers would continue to play a major role.

Under a public option, Americans would continue to have a choice of insurance plan, although their choice of provider could still be restricted by private insurance companies. The tax increases required to fund a public option would be far lower than those required for Medicare for All.

In a more fundamental sense, the public option would retain the consumer product model of health insurance. If a public option is added to our existing healthcare system, health insurance would remain a product sold in a marketplace and purchased by consumers. The difference is that one of those products would be sold by the government.

MEDICARE FOR SOME, PUBLIC OPTION FOR SOME

A final type of coverage expansion seeks to guarantee universal coverage while giving people a choice to obtain coverage from a private insurer. In essence, these reforms aim to combine universal coverage, rate-setting, and a public option.

One version of this is known as Medicare for America, named for a piece of legislation introduced in the US House of Representatives.[9] In essence, under this plan everyone who does *not* have insurance from their job would be automatically enrolled in Medicare—including people who are currently uninsured, who are on Medicaid, or who buy private insurance on the ACA marketplaces. Employers could choose between offering private insurance to their employees and moving all their employees onto the new version of Medicare. People whose employers offer private insurance would be given the choice between that insurance and Medicare. Job-based insurance would also face new regulations requiring coverage to become more comprehensive, and government would regulate the payment rates that providers would receive from private insurers. Current legislation would allow people enrolled in the new Medicare program to choose a private Medicare Advantage plan (discussed in more detail in the next section).

In essence, Medicare for America is a universal coverage system where most people are automatically enrolled in Medicare, and everyone else has a choice between Medicare and heavily regulated private insurance offered through employers. It could be looked at as Medicare for half, public option for half.

Medicare for America contains many of the same ingredients as Medicare for All. It achieves universal coverage. Coverage would become more comprehensive—both because Medicare itself would be made more comprehensive and because the government would require private insurance to become more comprehensive—although out-of-pocket costs would persist at moderate levels (in the most recent version of the legislation, out-of-pocket costs would be waived for households below 200 percent of the poverty line, and other households would have out-of-pocket costs capped according to a sliding scale that maxes out at $5,000 per year).[10] Medicare for America also extends the negotiating leverage of the federal government throughout the health system by allowing private insurers to benefit from public payment rates—essentially a version of all-payer rate-setting.

But there are significant differences. Medicare for America would retain the administrative complexity that costs hundreds of billions of dollars every year and creates large burdens for clinicians and patients to navigate. Out-of-pocket costs would be higher than in Medicare for All. Private insurance premiums would perpetuate the regressive financing that exists today. Finally, public accountability would be constrained, with private insurance companies continuing to play a large role in the health system—especially if private Medicare Advantage plans are included in the new program, as proposed in the most recent version of the legislation.

Under Medicare for America, many Americans would retain a choice of health insurance plan. However, it's not necessarily true that privately insured Americans could keep their current plan: new regulations would compel many private insurance plans to become more comprehensive, and employers could also decide unilaterally to move their employees into Medicare for America. The tax increases necessary to fund Medicare for America would also be significantly lower than those required for Medicare for All, primarily because many Americans would continue to pay private insurance premiums.

MEDICARE ADVANTAGE FOR ALL

Medicare Advantage for All is very similar to Medicare for America: people would be guaranteed coverage, with a choice between a public Medicare plan and a private Medicare Advantage plan. In terms of the three functions of health insurers, Medicare Advantage for All would be publicly financed through taxes, would have an option for private companies to manage the insurance, and would use publicly determined payment rates across the system.

Because Medicare Advantage is funded through taxes, it could be financed more progressively than Medicare for America, which maintains a larger role for regressive private insurance premiums. (This also means that Medicare Advantage for All would likely require tax increases similar to those for M4A.) But on the whole Medicare Advantage for All would be quite similar to Medicare for America, with both the attractions and challenges of maintaining a large role for private insurance companies.

Many of the reforms discussed in this chapter have never been tried at scale in the United States. But Medicare Advantage has already been implemented, where seniors can choose to exit the traditional Medicare program and instead get their coverage from a private Medicare Advantage plan. This provides real-world lessons for how a similar private option might function alongside an expanded Medicare program.

Supporters of Medicare Advantage hoped the program would decrease healthcare costs, based on the theory that private companies can manage insurance benefits more efficiently than a federal program. However, Advantage patients actually cost the government more than traditional Medicare patients.[11] Furthermore, Advantage plans have overhead costs nearly identical to the rest of the private insurance market: according to one estimate, Advantage plans spend 86 percent of premiums on medical care, with 14 percent left over for administrative costs and profits.[12] (Remember that traditional Medicare spends nearly 98 percent of its budget on medical care.)

A further difficulty is that Advantage plans attract healthier people, largely because healthier people are less bothered by the restrictions on care found in Advantage plans. Indeed, these restrictions can be effective tools to push the sickest patients out of Advantage plans: for instance, low-income seniors with high medical need quit their Advantage plans and return to traditional Medicare three to four times more frequently than their counterparts with fewer medical needs.[13] Because the government pays Advantage plans based on the costs of seniors in traditional Medicare, it's likely that the government is overpaying Advantage plans. The government tries to correct for this by paying Advantage plans less for healthier patients and more for sicker patients—but even when two seniors have the same health risk on paper, researchers have found that Advantage plans are still more likely to attract the person with lower medical spending.[14] The result is that though insurers get paid to cover people who are relatively sick, they are, in fact, covering people who are relatively healthy. Advantage plans use the windfall to expand benefits and boost their own profits, and taxpayers are left footing a higher bill. Advantage plans can also increase their profits by exaggerating how sick their enrollees look on paper in order to extract more payments from Medicare; indeed, in 2020 the Department of Justice sued both Cigna and Anthem alleging that their Advantage plans used this strategy to extract nearly $2 billion in fraudulent payments.[15] A final issue is that the proliferation of Advantage plans imposes an additional cost on doctors and hospitals, who must build up their administrative apparatus to interact with a multitude of payers with different rules and regulations.

A final consideration is that Advantage plans are appealing to many seniors today largely because they fill the gaps in the traditional Medicare plan: for instance, traditional Medicare has no out-of-pocket spending limit, prescription drug coverage must be purchased separately, and it doesn't offer dental, vision, and hearing benefits. If M4A is a truly comprehensive plan—with coverage for a wide range of benefits and minimal cost-sharing —the attraction of Medicare Advantage plans might be more limited.

COMPETITION AND SOLIDARITY

The plans just discussed—a public option, Medicare for America, and Medicare Advantage for All—differ in important ways. But they all feature a public insurance plan that "competes" with private plans, and people can choose for themselves which plan to carry. This raises an important technical challenge: for-profit health insurance companies don't *want* to insure unprofitable patients who require a lot of medical care. Instead of competing *for* the business of people with the greatest medical need, private insurers often compete to *turn them away*. This is the crux of our ongoing debate about preexisting conditions.

Insurers are no longer allowed to explicitly refuse coverage to people with preexisting conditions, but they can still deter sick patients using a variety of other techniques, like restricting provider networks, refusing to cover care from specialists who treat complex disorders, or excluding expensive medications from their list of covered drugs. (These strategies are nicknamed "cherry-picking" and "lemon-dropping.") According to one colorful exaggeration, "Insurers, like casinos, are profitable because they know the odds of every bet they take and can eject people who are beating the house."[16] Insurers can't remove particular individuals from their rolls, but it's true that insurance companies know which types of patients are losing them money and can try to minimize their enrollment. Indeed, bureaucratic "sludge" can be used as a deliberate strategy to cause the sickest patients to give up and switch into a plan with fewer restrictions on care, like the traditional Medicare program. As companies collect more and more of our personal data online and otherwise, the ability of insurance companies to engage in cherry-picking and lemon-dropping will only increase.

In contrast, a public option—which is accountable to voters rather than shareholders—is not likely to engage in these profit-maximizing tactics, instead welcoming all comers according to its social mission. The result is that sicker Americans are likely to be moved into the public option, while healthier enrollees will be cherry-picked by private insurance companies.

This sorting has serious consequences for healthcare costs. Because 5 percent of the population accounts for half of health spending in any given year, private insurers can benefit enormously by pushing the sickest Americans into the public plan.[17] The result is that the public plan is burdened with higher costs, and a two-tier system might develop where healthier and wealthier Americans are segregated from the rest of the population in terms of health insurance. Critics can then point to the higher costs in the public plan to argue that government is inefficient—even though the higher costs are a result of caring for patients with greater medical needs, whom private insurers don't want to cover.

A different kind of sorting can result when individual Americans are given the choice between paying a private insurance premium and paying for a public option. Public option proposals often set premiums according to a progressive schedule—for instance, Medicare for America would be free for people with incomes under 200 percent of the poverty line, with premiums increasing on a sliding scale until they max out at 8 percent of income for people with incomes above 600 percent of the poverty line. Regressive private insurance premiums work in exactly the opposite direction, with low-income people charged a higher proportion of income and high-income people charged a lower proportion. The result is that the public option would be more attractive for people who have less money, and private insurance would be more attractive for people who have more money.

This kind of segregation by income carries political risks. Public programs are more resilient when everyone has a stake in their success, including the wealthiest and most powerful members of society. It is much easier to threaten programs that disproportionately benefit the poor, like Medicaid. Universal programs like Medicare have more staying power.

CONCLUSION

The national health reform debate is filled with complex proposals. The technical details of these proposals are important. But too often, technical jargon is used to obscure the underlying values that a healthcare plan reflects.

At its core, the Affordable Care Act reflects a vision of healthcare as a regulated consumer product supported by a safety net. Proposals to strengthen the ACA continue this same vision while moving closer to universal coverage. On the cost side, market-based reforms are premised on the idea that we should try to make healthcare more like a typical competitive marketplace; in contrast, price regulation rests on the idea that market forces simply don't work well enough to control costs in healthcare.

Public option proposals share the basic vision of healthcare as a consumer product, except that one of the health insurance products available for purchase in the marketplace is offered by the government. This carries some important benefits, but the overall vision—healthcare as a regulated consumer product supported by a safety net—remains largely unchanged. An alternative vision is that the government should guarantee health insurance for all, but market forces and private insurance companies should retain a critical role; this is the goal of hybrid plans like Medicare for America and Medicare Advantage for All.

Medicare for All is the only proposal that seeks to fundamentally transform healthcare into a public good. In addition to the specific benefits it delivers—universal, comprehensive, cost-effective healthcare—Medicare for All should also be understood as a broader statement about social values.

When public values are in question, the debate necessarily moves into the political arena.

PART III

POLITICS

7
WE THE PEOPLE

Policy remains a matter of theory if it's not politically practicable—if there's no pathway to becoming law. Though the merits of the policy itself for the political potential of that policy, the process by which its merits are translated, picked apart, weighed, and measured is indirect at best. That process is a function of the power and political strategy of the coalitions that form in support of or opposition to it—and the light of the political moment in which it's being discussed.

Medicare for All has emerged as a defining point of discussion in our political discourse. That's probably why you're reading this book. In this section, we discuss the politics of M4A: how might M4A become law? In the light of history, we consider the current swell of support for M4A. What are the unique circumstances that have allowed it to become such a critical part of our healthcare discussion? Who constitutes the coalitions of people who support or oppose M4A, and why do they support or oppose it? Who's undecided? And what's the pathway for passage, if there is one?

Let's start with the most important stakeholder in health politics, we the people, and consider what may be shaping our attitudes toward M4A.

THE PEOPLE AND MEDICARE FOR ALL

There is one stakeholder in American healthcare that matters most: the American public. The public is, after all, the patient, the voter, and the taxpayer. And every other stakeholder in this debate, from the health insurance corporations to the grassroots organizers, seeks to change the public opinion.

Public support for M4A is high. A nationally representative Pew Research study found that most Americans agree "it is the responsibility of the federal government to make sure all Americans have health care coverage."[1] And a majority of Americans support M4A as a way to achieve this goal. In March 2018, the Kaiser Family Foundation asked 1,212 American adults, "Do you favor or oppose having a national health plan, or Medicare-for-all, in which all Americans would get their insurance from a single government plan?" Among all respondents, 59 percent were in favor and 38 percent were opposed.[2]

However, Americans are diverse—racially, demographically, socioeconomically, geographically, and politically.

And this diversity predictably shapes opinions about M4A. Politically, liberals and progressives have generally supported more government engagement with healthcare, while conservatives have opposed it—though there is some surprising support among Republicans. In November 2018, Politico and Morning Consult asked registered voters if they supported or opposed "a Medicare-for-all health system, where all Americans get their health insurance from the government," and found 58 percent total support, including 77 percent of Democrats, 60 percent of independents, and 41 percent of Republicans. (Notably, when the poll replaced the term "Medicare-for-all" with "single payer," support dropped from 58 percent to 49 percent overall.)[3] The majority of Democratic primary voters in 2020 said they preferred "a government plan for all instead of private insurance."[4]

Though geography maps closely to political preference, there is less geographic variation in support for M4A than you might expect. It's a common trope among centrist Democrats who oppose M4A to argue that it won't appeal to Americans in the "heartland." Here's Joe Donnelly, former Democratic senator for Indiana, for example: "When you talk Medicare for All . . . you lose people in my state."[5] But in fact, 55 percent of voters in Indiana support M4A, including presumably large majorities of Democrats. (Donnelly attacked M4A during his Senate reelection campaign in 2018, which he lost.) In total, an analysis of Kaiser Family Foundation data by Data for Progress estimated that a majority of voters support M4A in forty-two states.[6]

Generally, people of color are more likely to support M4A as well. A *New York Times* poll from November 2019 found that M4A was supported by 51 percent of white Americans, 60 percent of Hispanic Americans, and 70 percent of Black Americans.[7] Young people are also more likely to support M4A: 65 percent of people ages eighteen to thirty-four supported the policy, versus 42 percent of people fifty-five and older.

Wealthy Americans don't often have to deal with the holes in America's healthcare system, shielded by the security their wealth affords them. Meanwhile, poor Americans—including those who rely on Medicaid and those who are left in the gap between Medicaid and access to private insurance—are far more likely to experience the insecurity of falling off employer healthcare coverage due to losing a job, or the precariousness of trying to find a doctor who will take Medicaid. These experiences predictably shape perspectives on M4A: 64 percent of Americans making less than $50,000 a year support M4A, compared to 49 percent of those making over $100,000.[8]

Public support for M4A is high. But it hasn't always been this way. From 1998 to 2008, the Kaiser Family Foundation conducted ten polls asking Americans whether they supported a single-payer national health insurance program. None found majority support.[9] Between 2017 and May 2020, the same organization conducted fifteen similar polls. Every poll found majority support for M4A.[10]

WHY HAVE AMERICANS BECOME MORE SUPPORTIVE OF M4A?

It's a story of health insecurity and how to solve it. Prior to the economic crisis spurred by COVID-19, the Great Recession of 2007–9 was America's longest and deepest economic downturn since the Great Depression. As jobs went, so did health insurance, and more than 9 million Americans lost healthcare coverage during the Great Recession.[11] Those who did were disproportionately low-income, white, and living in the Midwest and South.[12] Losing healthcare has reverberating effects across entire communities. Watching a friend, neighbor, family member, or former colleague go through that experience can shape an individual's own perspective on healthcare security. The generation of children who watched their parents lose healthcare in the Great Recession is also coming of age today, which may contribute to the disproportionate support of M4A among young people. More broadly, the sudden loss of health security during the Great Recession may have planted seeds that help explain why support for M4A now crosses traditional geographic and ideological boundaries.

If that's the first piece of the story, the second is the saga of the Affordable Care Act. Following closely on the heels of the Great Recession, the ACA was meant to make healthcare coverage more secure. In many ways, it did. Twenty million Americans gained insurance. People with preexisting conditions were protected. People who didn't have coverage through their employer—like those who lost their jobs during the recession—now had more options for coverage.

But the political gamesmanship around the ACA has inflamed Americans' sense of healthcare insecurity. Although the calls to repeal and replace the ACA made it seem inevitable that the act would be dismantled after the 2016 elections, efforts to fully repeal the ACA were narrowly blocked. But that hasn't saved it from being sabotaged in other ways. These include expanding the availability of "short-term" plans that don't cover preexisting conditions and erecting new obstacles to enrollment—not to mention the lawsuit brought by twenty Republican state attorneys general that would undo the ACA's protections for preexisting conditions.

With every round of efforts to meddle with the ACA came a new round of public discussion and debate about what the consequences might be—a new round of forecasting about who might lose their healthcare, and how much healthcare costs might change. The constant droning of this debate raises consternation about healthcare security, forcing all but the most financially secure and healthy Americans to ask themselves if they would be okay. For a country collectively traumatized by the loss of healthcare less than a decade earlier, this has the effect of continuing to destabilize support for the current system in view of more secure alternatives.

The debate about preexisting conditions in the lead-up to the 2018 midterms accentuates this point: the GOP attacked these protections, and Democrats gained a net forty seats in the House.[13] Exit polling showed that a full 41 percent of voters identified healthcare as their primary concern coming into Election Day, and 57 percent of voters said that Democrats were the better party for people with preexisting conditions.[14]

But the most important piece in the story of healthcare insecurity and rising support for M4A may not be political at all. Simply put, job-based private insurance has eroded. In the decade after the Great Recession ended, premiums rose by 50 percent and deductibles doubled—though wages increased only 26 percent.[15] For a single person with employer coverage, by 2019 the average premium was $7,188 (nearly a fifth of which came directly from employees) to buy a plan with a $1,655 deductible.[16] That means a low-income worker might need to spend a full month's salary on out-of-pocket medical costs before insurance kicked in. Premiums for family coverage in 2019 exceeded $20,000. In certain plan types, average deductibles were nearly $5,000. As plans deteriorated, unexpected medical bills for uncovered services became both more common and more expensive.[17] The ACA got more people insured, but it did little to stop the fact that hospitals, doctors, and pharmaceutical companies were charging ever-higher prices to people with private insurance—driving premiums and deductibles so high that many Americans saw their coverage unravel.

People like Lisa Cardillo, whom we introduced in Chapter 1, became the collateral damage. Middle-class Americans like Lisa have been left in a precarious position, unsure if their health insurance will actually cover them when they need it most.

The COVID-19 pandemic accentuated these trends. At a time when people cared most about having adequate, secure healthcare in case they got sick, millions of Americans lost their jobs, and with them their health insurance. A study from the non-partisan advocacy group Families USA estimated that 5.4 million laid-off workers became uninsured between February and May of 2020.[18]

Loss of health security appears to be driving support for M4A. Compared with people who favor building on the ACA, Americans who favor M4A report that they are less satisfied with their current health insurance coverage, less satisfied with their ability to get healthcare when they need it, less satisfied with the cost of their healthcare, and more worried about being able to pay their medical bills if they get sick.[19] They are also more likely to have a negative view of employer-provided private insurance. When Americans get hurt by our healthcare system, they're more likely to turn toward M4A for relief. Indeed, in the midst of the COVID-19 pandemic, support for M4A jumped to a nine-month high.[20]

Lisa put it simply: "I feel like if you've been in the situation that we've been in, you would be for Medicare for All."

The perspective of middle-class Americans like Lisa will be critical to the M4A debate. According to Rashi Fein, an American economist who helped develop Medicare, "Only when the broad middle class is being hurt and when it becomes clear that private solutions will not suffice—as in the case of Social Security and Medicare—does America turn to universal programs addressed to all its citizens."[21] Reflecting on the failure of national health insurance in the 1970s, Fein concluded that "for most Americans that time had not yet come."

As we enter the third decade of the twenty-first century, the time may have come when the broad middle class is being hurt by our healthcare system—and many are beginning to question whether private health insurance will suffice to alleviate the pain.

The final piece of the story, which we'll discuss in more detail in Chapter 10, is the emergence of a grassroots movement allied with political leaders like Senator Bernie Sanders and Representative Alexandria Ocasio-Cortez that sought to orient the growing unease around health insecurity toward a policy prescription: M4A.

The Terms of the Debate

Americans want health security. Finding themselves paying more for insurance that covers less, they are increasingly coming to view M4A as a stable, secure alternative to the status quo. At the same time, opponents to M4A have sought to frame their opposition to M4A around healthcare security as well. In that respect, our public discussion about M4A reflects opposing arguments about how M4A could either provide Americans healthcare security or erode it.

Though public support for M4A is high, some commentators think this support is an illusion. "It's candy," one political veteran told us. "People like candy, people will take candy, people will consume candy. But then as soon as you realize that there's some sour spice in the candy, then you're going to think twice . . . If you just stick your finger in it and give people some easy, negative arguments about it, the support diminishes rapidly."

Is support for M4A really so fickle? Let's take a look at the major arguments that opponents have deployed to attack M4A: it will take away your insurance, it will raise your taxes, it's a government takeover of healthcare, and the transition will take away jobs and leave people without healthcare.

The first attack is simple: "M4A will take away your private health insurance." Of course, M4A would also *give* you comprehensive health insurance for life. But that's why this attack is so ingenious: it invokes the fear of health insecurity as an argument *against* guaranteed healthcare. This attack might be especially potent for privately-insured Americans who are healthy enough not to have had to use their insurance in the past—though likely less so for people like Lisa, who have had to rely on it and found it wanting.

Even if M4A would be better than private insurance, *losing* anything isn't something people look forward to. John McDonough, a public health professor who worked on the ACA, told us, "People, by nature, fear hypothetical losses more than they appreciate hypothetical gains. So if I say to one person, 'I'm going to take $5 from you,' and if I say to another person, 'I'm going to give you $5,' the person who I tell I'm going to give them something says, 'I'll believe it when I see it.' And the person who believes that I might actually try to take it will hang on to their wallet and get their switchblade ready for me when I come after them."

The attack has been effective. Polls have considered whether, in follow-up questions, people reverse their support for M4A when they are told they would need to give up their private health insurance. One poll from the Kaiser Family Foundation in November 2019 found that support for M4A dipped from 53 percent to 37 percent when respondents were told it would "eliminate private health insurance companies."[22] Avoiding this vulnerability is a principal reason many of the alternatives to M4A, which we discussed in Chapter 6, focus specifically on allowing people to keep their private health insurance.

People are understandably concerned about losing their healthcare. But are they worried about losing their insurance company or about losing their healthcare providers? The same Kaiser poll quoted above explored this question, telling respondents that M4A would "eliminate private health insurance, but allow people to choose their doctors, hospitals, and other medical providers." Support more than rebounded, back up to 54 percent.[23] Public opinion on M4A may be malleable, but it is not fickle.

The second major attack against M4A is that it would raise taxes. As discussed in Part II of this book, M4A is likely to reduce healthcare costs for the vast majority of Americans. However, while the cost of the current healthcare system comes in the form of premiums extracted automatically from a biweekly or monthly paycheck—and then a host of out-of-pocket costs at the point of care—M4A would be funded with new progressive taxes.

Pundits have often oversimplified the story on this issue: "People love Medicare for All until they're told it'll raise their taxes," as one headline put it.[24] This claim is based on another Kaiser poll, which found that support dropped to 37 percent if people were told M4A would require most Americans to pay more in taxes.[25] But Americans have proven to be more sophisticated than the skeptics assume. When the same pollsters asked for people's views if M4A would "increase the taxes you personally pay, but decrease your overall costs for healthcare," support rebounded to 47 percent in favor, 48 percent opposed.[26] Other polls specifically tested support for a Medicare for All plan financed without new taxes on the middle class (an option described in Chapter 5), finding 57 percent support vs. 30 percent opposition.[27]

There's no doubt that taxes are a vulnerability for M4A, but it may not be the Achilles' heel that skeptics fear.

The third major line of attack is that M4A will entrust healthcare to a government bureaucracy. A popular meme is to point to long lines for government services like at the post office or the Department of Motor Vehicles and argue that M4A would bring these waiting lines to healthcare—"If you like the DMV, you'll love Medicare for All," in the words of one Republican congressman.[28] But whether post office lines are too long is really beside the point: these attacks deliberately misrepresent the role of government under M4A, evoking an image of overcrowded government facilities rather than private hospitals and clinics accessed by people with publicly funded insurance.

Similarly, opponents argue that M4A would force healthcare rationing. Of course, this attack ignores the fact that our *current* system rations healthcare—though instead of it being rationed by need, it is rationed by income. Despite the fearmongering about "government rationing," Medicare itself guarantees access to care that often exceeds what's available with private insurance. (In practical terms, what is and is not covered under M4A—and the process by which these decisions are made—may emerge as a key consideration for those concerned about rationing and increased government involvement.)

A fourth, more targeted line of attack focuses on the transition to M4A. Estimates suggest that more than 800,000 people work in the private health insurance industry—and that M4A might cost many of them their jobs.[29] Furthermore, transitioning to M4A on a two- or four-year timeline would create a window of deep insecurity. Considering the federal government's botched rollout of HealthCare.gov, how can we trust the government to execute a mass transition to government health insurance competently? And finally, considering Republican efforts to repeal the ACA, some Democrats argue that leaving M4A in Republican hands could spell disaster for the healthcare of millions of Americans.

Though the transition to M4A may cost health insurance industry jobs, this line of attack ignores the fact that M4A also stands to generate a tremendous number of new healthcare jobs by reintroducing tens of millions of Americans into the healthcare system. Furthermore, much of the administration of M4A would still fall to insurance professionals, albeit ones who are working for the government or government contractors rather than for private for-profit corporations. Furthermore, while the rollout of M4A would be an immense undertaking, most plans articulate a staged approach, allowing lessons learned at each stage to improve the next stage. And finally, like Social Security and Medicare itself, the ACA was never actually repealed. That's because in the history of American politics, it's been nearly impossible to repeal universal entitlements—once Americans have them, they choose overwhelmingly to keep them. So while some Republican administrations might be tempted to try, they know that attempting to repeal M4A would likely portend disaster at the polls.

The back-and-forth over these issues—losing insurance, raising taxes, government control, and the transition to M4A—certainly matters for public opinion. M4A supporters have effective responses to these charges: you'd keep your doctor and switch to more comprehensive insurance, most people would pay less for healthcare, and it'd work like Medicare today. But which side of the story will Americans hear? More broadly, if public conversation is focused on these issues, it means the opponents of M4A have already succeeded in framing the debate. It means we're *not* focused on the core issues facing healthcare today: that it is unaffordable, too many people are priced out, Americans are living shorter and sicker lives, and the experience of giving and receiving care is eroding.

In other words, the battle for public opinion is not just a contest of ideas. It's also a contest of power, with supporters and opponents deploying all the resources at their disposal to get their message in front of people and change hearts and minds. For nearly a century, the well-funded industry opponents of universal healthcare have leveraged negative advertising to get their message out on television, on the radio, in print, and now online and over social media. More importantly, they have used this negative advertising to frame the debate in ways that influence the broader discussion we have about health reform—whether in news articles, on talk shows, around the water cooler at work, or in text messages with friends. Indeed, many of the alternatives to M4A outlined in the previous chapter are partly designed to avert these negative attacks: some alternatives try to avoid the ire of the healthcare industry entirely, and others try to avoid the specific charges of taking away people's insurance, raising people's taxes, or unleashing a "government takeover of healthcare." Some proposals attempt to capture the rhetorical appeal of M4A by keeping the "Medicare for" moniker but hope that a less disruptive plan will prevent opponents from pushing the debate onto ruinous terrain. However, *any* plan to expand Medicare and reduce the price of healthcare is likely to draw the ire of industry, and the Affordable Care Act debates make clear that extreme rhetorical attacks can be used against even incremental plans. Rather than trying to avoid attacks from industry, the strategy for supporters of M4A must be to overcome them.

The lesson is that public opinion toward M4A does not exist in a vacuum. It will be deeply influenced by the coalitions lined up on either side of the debate—and by how they flex their power.

8
FOR AND AGAINST

Organized interest groups have played a powerful role in both the successes and failures of health reform throughout American history. Doctors led a startlingly effective attack campaign against Harry Truman's national health insurance plan in the 1940s, and insurance companies followed suit in the 1990s to tank Bill Clinton's healthcare plan. In contrast, the Affordable Care Act succeeded in large part because it was able to win the support of the healthcare industry. Medicare is perhaps the lone example in American history of major health reform that passed despite broad opposition from healthcare interest groups, buoyed instead by seniors and the labor movement.

As with prior reform efforts, the prospects of M4A—and the political strategy that might be deployed to get it passed—will depend critically on the stakeholders that are lined up for and against the proposal.

Healthcare interest groups have two central aims when attempting to impact major legislative debates: to shape public opinion, and to influence political campaigns and elected officials. In turn, there are at least three types of resources these groups deploy in pursuit of their influence: money, trust, and people power. Money can be used to fund media campaigns, lobbying efforts, and campaign contributions. Trust (and expertise, which is often invoked to establish trust) can be leveraged to influence the opinions of politicians and the public. People power can be deployed for direct activism and advocacy, can be used to build public support through personal conversations, and can be translated into votes for electoral victories. The political battle over M4A will depend largely on how competing stakeholders utilize their money, trust, and people power on both sides of the debate. Here we explore who those stakeholders are, where they stand on M4A (and why), and how they'll engage with the M4A debate.

SUPPORTING MEDICARE FOR ALL: NURSES AND OTHER HEALTHCARE PROVIDERS

With the decline in physician power and the growth of team-based healthcare, there has been a rise in the power of healthcare providers other than doctors. In part this is because the past several decades have seen a rapid expansion in physician assistants and nurse practitioners, and in part because of powerful nurses and medical staff unions that have emerged since the mid-twentieth century.

Nurses and other front-line clinical workers have become powerful voices in support of M4A. One of the strongest and most effective advocates for M4A in the country is National Nurses United (NNU), organizing over 150,000 nurses nationwide. Their influence nationally as well as locally, through the organizing efforts of their state branches, has helped elevate M4A in the national debate. Similarly, the Service Employees International Union (SEIU), with over 2 million members including home care workers, doctors, nurses, and other medical staff, has emerged as another important voice in the healthcare debate that supports M4A. Given that nurses and medical staff vastly outnumber doctors, it is natural that they have gained a strong voice in the health reform debate.

One reason behind the growing support of M4A among nurses and allied health professionals is the growth and consolidation of major healthcare corporations. As their employers grow in power, nurses and allied health professionals face a reduction in bargaining leverage, as oligopolies can tighten ranks regarding union contract terms with respect to pay, overtime, and staffing ratios. Healthcare workers' unions see M4A as a step to regaining negotiating power. Furthermore, unions could lobby a government single payer to mandate safer staffing ratios and collective bargaining rights: for instance, HR1384 (the M4A bill in the House) indicates that a Medicare for All program could set national minimum standards for healthcare institutions, including safe staffing ratios.

Furthermore, nurses enter the healthcare debate not only as healthcare professionals but also as members of the American middle class who face the same struggles with health insurance as their peers in other lines of work. Finally, all healthcare providers face growing demands on their time, imposed on them by a fragmented and inefficient healthcare system, and they see firsthand how that system harms patients on a daily basis. Their support for M4A is founded in their advocacy for their patients and for themselves.

These healthcare workers leverage two critical sources of power. First, they are a reputable and trusted arbiter of healthcare interests for the general public—indeed, nurses have been ranked the most trusted professionals in America for eighteen years straight.[1] Second, their unions are potent sources of people power. They are among the most adept and committed organizers in the healthcare debate, helping organize people and resources to broaden support and engage in direct activism.

SUPPORTING MEDICARE FOR ALL: PROGRESSIVE GRASSROOTS ADVOCACY ORGANIZATIONS

The progressive movement has taken up M4A as one of its flagship causes, providing a strong coalition of dedicated, organized, and effective groups in support of M4A. They include progressive civic action organizations like Amnesty International, the League of Women Voters, and the National

Association for the Advancement of Colored People, as well as grassroots organizations on the left, such as the Center for Popular Democracy, Public Citizen, Social Security Works, Democratic Socialists of America, Indivisible, the Women's March, and the Working Families Party. And they include think tanks like Demos as well as faith organizations like the United Methodist Church, Presbyterian Church, and Unitarian Universalist Church.

These organizations operate as critical local conveners and organizers, canvassing their communities and driving pressure on local and national elected officials. They lead on the tactical approach to organizing, leveraging their local clout to help build the coalition necessary to drive change. They are also critical to helping elect progressive, pro-M4A representatives to office.

Representative Ro Khanna, a progressive supporter of M4A from Northern California, illustrated how influential these grassroots organizations can be. He told us: "We've got mobilized citizens across the country. . . . You've had groups like Democracy for America, the Progressive Change Campaign Committee, MoveOn, Our Revolution, that have made the case for M4A—for a single-payer system—and then now you have citizen activists everywhere who understand that this is the best way to reduce costs, and also to give everyone the healthcare that they need." He's seen the grassroots energy firsthand: "I know in my town halls that the majority of questions when we're discussing issues are about healthcare. I often get the loudest applause when I talk about my support for Bernie Sanders and Pramila Jayapal's new Medicare for All bills."

These grassroots organizers will be the hub of people power in support of M4A. Their ability to leverage new organizing techniques to draw attention to the case for M4A and shift policymaker perspectives is critical to passing M4A, as we'll explore more in Chapter 10.

AGAINST MEDICARE FOR ALL: HEALTHCARE CORPORATIONS

In almost every reform effort, there was one incredibly powerful voice that opposed reform, whether it was Truman's national health insurance plan or the Clinton-era reform efforts: Big Healthcare.

The most important and most powerful opposition to M4A is healthcare corporations. Indeed, they are by far the most powerful lobbying interest in American healthcare—and among the most powerful in American politics writ large.[2] Over the last two decades the pharmaceutical industry and the insurance industry have been the number one and number two biggest spenders on lobbying in the entire country, putting up about $4 billion and $3 billion, respectively, over that period.[3] Hospitals and nursing homes came in at number eight, spending almost $2 billion. In terms of individual lobbying organizations, Big Healthcare consistently has three groups in the nation's top six—Pharmaceutical Research and Manufacturers of America, Blue Cross Blue

Shield, and the American Hospital Association, which together spent almost twice as much in 2019 than Amazon, Facebook, and Google combined.[4]

These healthcare corporations have grown in size and gone down in number. Because of major growth in the insurance and pharmaceutical industries and the massive consolidation discussed earlier, they became even more powerful in the latter half of the twentieth century. For example, consolidation of hospital systems has occurred at breakneck speed, and more than 60 percent of community hospitals in the United States now belong to a health system.[5] Estimates suggest that in the next decade, consolidation will consume 50 percent of currently operating health systems.[6]

Within the healthcare ecosystem, consolidation has increased the power of administrators in those systems over the health professionals they employ. Between 1975 and 2010, the number of physicians grew 150 percent. During the same time frame, the number of health administrators grew 3,200 percent.[7] This class of administrators, largely speaking for and with the growing healthcare corporations they represent, has become a powerful stakeholder in American healthcare.

Across the board, these healthcare corporations oppose M4A. For insurers, M4A is an existential threat to business as they know it. Indeed, a central purpose of M4A is to guarantee comprehensive insurance to all, without the need for private insurance companies.

The pharmaceutical industry opposes M4A because it would likely empower the federal government to negotiate the price of prescription drugs—the single most important concern for the industry.

Elected officials are clear about how powerful these industries can be. Representative Khanna was straightforward with us: "The insurance industry and Big Pharma will be the biggest opposition."

Most hospital corporations are likely to oppose M4A as well. Leveraging lucrative contracts from private insurers is critical to their strategy of growth and profit. M4A would give the government the power to set the rates paid to even the most powerful hospitals and would eliminate the collusion between large hospitals and large insurers that has made the winners of consolidation very rich.

John McDonough, the public health professor who worked on ACA reform, echoed the idea that hospitals would go to battle to prevent any decline in reimbursement. He told us that if the local hospital "is getting on average 180 percent of Medicare rates [from private insurers], and you're telling them that you're going to bring them down to 110 percent or 120 percent . . . I mean, they'll run you out of the room with pitchforks." (To clarify: private insurance payments account for about 40 percent of hospital revenue on average, and M4A would have the leverage to bring down payment rates for those patients.[8] As discussed in Chapter 4, M4A would benefit hospitals in other ways that could partly or wholly offset this change, with the impact varying widely across different hospitals.)

Further, M4A might alter the allocation of healthcare spending across providers. For instance, it might incentivize primary care over specialty care to help alleviate the primary care shortage, or it might equalize payments to healthcare facilities in currently under-resourced rural and urban communities. This could disrupt current lines of business, especially for the wealthiest providers. Finally, M4A also has the potential to empower the labor side of healthcare against the systems they work in, reducing corporate profits still more.

It's important to note that there is a cadre of hospitals who are less opposed to M4A, including safety net and nonprofit hospitals that serve low-income populations. In general, these are the hospitals that have been left behind over the past several decades as richer systems have consolidated and soaked up resources. The CEO of UMass Memorial Health Care, which operates multiple hospitals in central Massachusetts, said, "[Wealthier] organizations generally oppose Medicare for All because they oppose the prospect of reducing commercial rates down to Medicare rates. By contrast, safety net hospitals should consider Medicare for All as an opportunity to be more fairly reimbursed for treating those patients who are central to their missions—i.e., those who are either uninsured or covered by Medicaid."[9] He said M4A could help "level the playing field between the hospitals that take care of the poor people and hospitals that take care of the rich people."[10] Representative Pramila Jayapal, lead sponsor of HR1384, noted another such example: "I remember [a] children's hospital coming in to see us and they were not closed to it at all. In fact, they were really excited about the idea that kids would be able to get whatever care they needed."

But money talks: the wealthiest hospitals who have the most to lose under M4A also tend to be the most powerful. Unsurprisingly, the American Hospital Association is adamantly opposed to M4A.

Hospitals might prove to be an especially potent foe. The giant hospital systems formed over the last several decades have yet to show their full might as opponents to major health reform, having been won over early on in the effort to pass the Affordable Care Act. Hospital revenue is over $1 trillion per year—nearly 5 percent of GDP—and the collective might of the industry cannot be underestimated.

Hospitals also have two resources that insurance and pharmaceutical companies lack: local power and public trust. Insurance and pharmaceutical corporations have their headquarters clustered in places like New Jersey and Connecticut, but they don't have a local presence in many communities across the nation. In contrast, hospitals are the number one employer in many congressional districts, giving them special influence on members of the House. Furthermore, politicians are more comfortable making public enemies of insurance companies and Big Pharma, businesses that don't usually engender much public affection—indeed, the pharmaceutical industry is rated as the most disliked sector in the entire economy.[11] But the local hospital that cared for your sick relative? Harder to demonize. Hospitals are banking on that trust in the fight against M4A. "Right now, some person that is uninsured . . . comes to our ER, we take care of them," explains the president of the New York hospital lobby. "How in the name of God are you going to criticize that?"[12]

More broadly, major healthcare corporations have huge stockpiles of cash—the proceeds of the most expensive healthcare system in the world. They leverage that money to move the public conversation by maxing out on campaign contributions, supporting industry-friendly candidates with outside spending during elections, hiring armies of lobbyists on Capitol Hill, and launching massive advertising campaigns to sway public opinion.

AGAINST MEDICARE FOR ALL: THE CONSERVATIVE INFRASTRUCTURE

Since 2018, the Republican Party has made opposition to M4A a central part of its position on healthcare. Unable to repeal the ACA and suffering a stinging rebuke in the 2018 midterm elections resulting in part from their opposition to it, and without a clear alternative, Republicans have fixated on opposing M4A as both "socialized medicine" and a "government takeover" of healthcare. Because they have staked so much of their position on healthcare as being against M4A, it is exceedingly unlikely that any elected Republican will support M4A in the foreseeable future—even if a significant minority of Republican voters are open to the idea. M4A also threatens traditional conservative values of small government and low taxes (even if many conservative groups staunchly support the existing Medicare program).

For all these reasons, the full conservative infrastructure has lined up against M4A, including the Republican National Committee; advocacy organizations like Turning Point USA, FreedomWorks, and the American Action Network; and conservative think tanks like the Heritage Foundation, the American Legislative Exchange Center, and the Mercatus Center. These organizations are already investing deeply in anti-M4A efforts. Industry opponents of M4A provide critical funding to these conservative groups, including multimillion-dollar donations from the pharmaceutical and insurance industries.[13]

The Coalition Against Socialized Medicine is one of the networks organizing conservative opposition to M4A. Their website quotes Vladimir Lenin that "socialized medicine is the keystone to the arch of a socialist state"—the exact same (apparently fabricated) quote used by the American Medical Association to tarnish Truman's national health plan nearly eighty years ago.[14]

The conservative infrastructure will come at M4A with all three major sources of power. Their network of think tanks has already begun to coordinate the argument against M4A. They are spending on extensive advertising campaigns to move their message. Finally, they have a strong network of grass-tops organizations—well-funded organizations designed to look and feel like grassroots groups to mobilize people power—that can organize in opposition to M4A, and they are hoping that the opportunity to defeat "socialism" will motivate their base to turn out to the polls.

AGAINST MEDICARE FOR ALL: THE CENTRIST DEMOCRATIC INFRASTRUCTURE

Many centrist Democratic leaders are intensely skeptical of M4A and hope to prevent it from becoming the Democratic Party's standard position on healthcare. To be sure, some of these leaders would genuinely prefer to live in a world governed by the Affordable Care Act or one of the alternative reform plans detailed in Chapter 6 rather than M4A. But in large part their opposition is a political judgment: they fear that Democrats will suffer electoral defeat if the party unites behind M4A, and that a major legislative push for M4A would end in failure.

Much of this opposition stems from veterans of previous battles for healthcare reform during the Clinton and Obama eras who recall the pain and consequences of the fierce opposition they faced in the past. Further, they argue that the path to victory—to improving healthcare coverage—runs through the middle of the electorate, and that M4A is too far left, an extreme idea that will lose centrist Democrats and independents.

Opposition to M4A based on political strategy often bleeds into substantive attacks on M4A as a policy. Especially for political leaders, it's not very exciting to say, "Medicare for All is good policy but I don't think we can get it done." It's more compelling to argue that M4A is wrong on the merits and your alternative proposal is better. The result is that some centrist Democrats deploy many of the same talking points used by Republican opponents and the healthcare industry—M4A will throw you off your insurance, raise your taxes, take away your choice, and cost jobs—sowing further doubts about whether M4A is a wise direction for reform. For their part, industry opponents of M4A support the campaigns of these more centrist Democrats and try to defeat progressive Democrats who endorse M4A. Industry support of centrist candidates leaves progressives with an electoral disadvantage regardless of the popularity of their platform among voters.

Tactically, centrist Democratic leaders who oppose M4A use their public platforms to make the political and substantive case against M4A. The broader Democratic establishment also leverages the trust they've engendered through supporting and defending the Affordable Care Act since the Obama years. In proposing alternative health reforms, they rely on the work of center-left think tanks like the Center for American Progress, Third Way, and the Progressive Policy Institute. Because the vast majority of Democratic voters support M4A, these groups have limited ability to organize people power against M4A.

9

STAKEHOLDERS IN FLUX

Though there are clear supporters and opponents of Medicare for All, there are also critical stakeholders in healthcare politics who have not yet firmly aligned for or against the reform. That's largely because these groups aren't yet certain how M4A would affect them. This is where policy and politics collide: the positions of these swing constituencies will depend partly on the policy choices we examined in Chapter 4.

Still, the material impact that a policy is projected to have on a group is only one factor determining whether that group will ultimately support or oppose it. Policy substance also interacts in complex ways with issues of identity, values, framing, trust, process, and history. Policy can help build a coalition, but it is no replacement for organizing. Ideally, political leaders can fuse policy *with* organizing, working collaboratively with stakeholders to craft policy they can organize their members around.

The key swing constituencies on M4A are doctors, labor unions, seniors, and large and small businesses. Will they join Big Healthcare, the conservative infrastructure, and centrist Democratic leaders in opposing M4A? Or will they join front-line clinical workers and the progressive movement in supporting it? Their decisions will have profound consequences for the money, trust, and people power deployed in the M4A debate to shape public opinion and influence the political process.

PHYSICIANS

Physicians have historically been a critical stakeholder in health reform debates. As discussed in Chapter 2, the American Medical Association played a central role in fighting previous attempts at national health insurance, especially the Truman plan and Medicare. But both physician preferences and power may be changing fast. Most individual physicians today support M4A. The *New England Journal of Medicine* surveyed clinicians and found that 55 percent supported single-payer healthcare.[1] (Note, however, that only 39 percent of healthcare executives supported it.)[2] A similar poll by Merritt Hawkins, a consulting firm, found that 56 percent of clinicians sampled supported single-payer healthcare.[3]

But the most vocal opposition to healthcare reform has traditionally come through physician organizations, like the

AMA. That, too, is changing. The AMA has historically been the dominant voice for American doctors, but the organization has lost clout over the past several decades. In the mid-twentieth century, nearly three in four physicians were members of the AMA. That membership has declined sharply: as of 2011, only about 15 percent of practicing physicians were members.[4] Still, the AMA remains the most powerful lobbying body of American physicians. The AMA is consistently among the top ten highest-spending lobbying groups in the nation; in 2019, it spent over $20 million on lobbying, ranking above Amazon and Facebook.

The AMA is at a crossroads regarding its stance on health reform. It broke with tradition to support the health coverage expansion of the Affordable Care Act. However, it was also quick to voice support for Tom Price, President Trump's first pick for Secretary of Health and Human Services and himself a physician, who was supposed to lead efforts to repeal the Affordable Care Act. In terms of national health insurance, in its 2017 vision statement on health reform the AMA neither supported nor opposed M4A.[5] But comments from AMA leadership have been less supportive: in October 2018, the president of the AMA told reporters that M4A would break her medical practice because government payment rates are too low.[6] More pointedly, the AMA was a founding member of the anti-M4A lobbying group known as the Partnership for America's Healthcare Future—though the AMA later left the group, following protests from its members and others in the medical profession.

Within the AMA, medical students and younger doctors have engaged in an active effort to pull the AMA's position toward M4A. Their efforts are showing signs of progress: in June 2019, the AMA's House of Delegates voted on a resolution to drop its opposition to single-payer healthcare, which only narrowly failed, garnering 47 percent of votes.[7]

There are also a handful of important physician organizations with an explicit focus on patient advocacy, including Doctors for America, the National Physicians Alliance, and Physicians for a National Health Program (PNHP). The last of these specifically advocates for single-payer healthcare and has worked diligently to keep this issue in the reform conversation since the 1980s. Indeed, the original M4A bill introduced in 2003—the Expanded and Improved Medicare for All Act (HR676)—was based on PNHP's "Physicians' Proposal for a National Health Program."

As the AMA's dominance has waned, medical societies organized around particular medical specialties have grown. For example, the American College of Physicians—the nation's largest group of doctors after the AMA—and similar groups represent over 350,000 primary care physicians.[8] In a historic shift, in early 2020 the American College of Physicians endorsed single-payer healthcare as an option to achieve universal coverage. The American Medical Student Association has also endorsed M4A, another signal that the profession may be evolving.

Why have physicians started warming to M4A? One reason is the increasingly onerous administrative burden that the private insurance system has imposed on doctors. Because each insurance company has its own billing criteria, billing forms, and billing requirements—in addition to its own rules for what services and medications are covered—the administrative overhead that physicians face is extraordinary. Estimates suggest that about one-sixth of a physician's work burden is attributable to administrative overhead in the multiple-payer environment we have today.[9] Physicians are beginning to recognize that a single-payer system might reduce this burden and facilitate their core work of treating patients. Furthermore, physicians' historical opposition to national health insurance has been based in part on a desire to prevent intrusion into the physician-patient relationship. But now that the insurance industry has penetrated so deeply into clinical care, many physicians are starting to see single-payer as a better alternative.

A second major reason is the changing nature of physician employment. For the vast majority of American medical history, most physicians worked in private practices that were owned by other physicians. Under this model, physicians would vest in ownership stakes in their own practice and over time become partners. This partnership model allowed doctors to control the businesses in which they worked, giving doctors a powerful voice in the business of healthcare. But over the past several decades, physicians have generally lost power and autonomy in the healthcare setting because of the growth and consolidation of major health systems. A 2017 representative survey of doctors found, for the first time, that the average doctor no longer owns her own practice.[10] More important is that younger doctors are less likely than older ones to work in physician-owned practices, signaling a generational shift in physician practice norms. This has serious implications for physician political power: more doctors are now employees of large healthcare corporations, rather than employees of other doctors.

For doctors, this has meant that being a physician no longer means being a business owner, as more of the means of production in healthcare are consolidated by the healthcare corporations. Physicians are beginning to see M4A as a way of keeping independent practices viable in the face of consolidation (as described in Part II). And with many physicians now employed and paid directly by a healthcare corporation, publicly administered payment rates may be perceived to have less of an impact on their personal finances.

During the COVID-19 pandemic, many large hospital systems struggled to provide basic personal protective equipment (PPE) and other supplies to physicians on the front lines. And when physicians sought to sound the alarm or obtain PPE outside their hospitals, some were silenced or even dismissed.[11] In this way the pandemic threw into sharp relief many of the trends driving doctors toward M4A, including the growing recognition that practicing physicians have interests that are separate from (and sometimes at odds with) the interests of the healthcare corporations that increasingly employ them.

There are also notable differences of opinion across medical specialties. Compared to primary care doctors, pediatricians, or infectious disease specialists, those practicing in the most lucrative specialties (like orthopedic surgery or neurosurgery) are less likely to support M4A. Specialties that can use the threat of surprise billing to collect higher fees, like radiologists and emergency physicians, could also see M4A as hazardous to their earnings (not to mention the private equity firms that have helped pioneer surprise billing as a business strategy). Medical student debt also remains an important source of insecurity for young physicians concerned about potential changes in compensation resulting from M4A.

Changing views toward M4A reflect a broader shift in the political orientation of physicians as well. Throughout the 1990s, physicians contributed twice as much to Republicans as they did to Democrats; by 2018, those numbers had reversed.[12] This swing reflects two facts: more Americans with advanced degrees have shifted to the Democratic Party, and more women and people of color (who lean Democratic) have entered medicine.

Finally, burnout is high among doctors. When the health system interferes with doctors' principal work of providing healthcare to people, they are left to navigate the consequences. As reviewed in Chapter 1, there are many problems with the system as it stands, and few are as brutal or alarming as the lack of access to healthcare that too many Americans have to face. Providers on the front lines meet these people, see their faces, hear their stories, and know their names. And for many health providers, beyond the relative bargaining power they might accrue or the administrative burdens they might avoid, the driver of their potential support for M4A is the notion that no patient—no person—would have to go without healthcare in the future.

Representative Pramila Jayapal, lead sponsor of HR1384, said: "Five years ago, physicians were not necessarily with us. But as people have gotten more and more frustrated with having to advocate with the insurance company on behalf of their patient, I think they've gotten very, very frustrated at how much time they're spending doing that and how little time they're spending doing the thing they actually went to school to do: provide quality care."

Doctors are critical because alongside nurses, they remain the most trusted arbiter of what's best for patients. As the front line of the healthcare system for the American public, they interact daily with the people they treat, providing a natural space for education and advocacy—even organizing—during national health reform debates.

Given changes in the power and preferences of physicians, doctors are a key swing constituency that could emerge as an important ally of M4A—or join the bloc of industry opposition.

There are several critical policy decisions that could influence physician support for M4A. They relate to physician payment, medical liability insurance, and medical education costs and debt.

One of the key reasons physicians may oppose M4A is financial. On average, physicians are able to negotiate 40 percent higher reimbursements from private insurers than they receive from Medicare.[13] Furthermore, reimbursement rates are quite variable by specialty and location. One veteran of the Obama-era reform efforts told us, "You might get the pediatricians and the family physicians on your side, you know, a few of the lower-paid groups. And the rest will kill you."

Beyond the value of reimbursement is *how* reimbursement is done. HR1384, for example, offers global payments—payments to healthcare institutions on a quarterly basis to cover all the care they are to provide for the next quarter. Giving the full budget for care to health system administrators could further shift control away from clinicians, and hospitals may try to squeeze the providers and provider groups they currently contract with to care for patients. In that respect, physician support for M4A may turn on how reimbursement rates are determined and how they compare to current rates. Aside from reimbursement, M4A legislation could consider additional provider protections to garner physician support, like setting guidelines for work hours or guaranteeing that clinicians can share in a portion of the revenue earned by the institutions that employ them.

Another policy consideration is malpractice liability. Though best estimates suggest that physician malpractice accounts for only 1–2 percent of overall healthcare costs, the fear of malpractice litigation is a significant nuisance for most physicians.[14] In a national survey of physicians in 2017, more than half reported having been involved in malpractice lawsuits.[15] Of those involved, 87 percent were taken by surprise and 89 percent felt the suit was unwarranted. And 81 percent said that they practice medicine with the threat of malpractice on their minds—a threat that influences behavior among 73 percent of those sampled.

Medical liability costs tend to be substantially lower in countries with single-payer healthcare.[16] Under M4A, one opportunity to build support among physicians would be to offer malpractice insurance through Medicare. In Canada, for example, nearly 95 percent of physicians are covered by the Canadian Medical Protective Association, which is a nonprofit organization established by the Parliament of Canada that indemnifies its members against damages and legal fees. Under M4A, such a service could be offered directly by Medicare, taking the burden of this nuisance off physicians.

Another potential policy lever is the cost of medical education, which is extremely expensive in the United States. More than three-fourths of medical students graduate with debt. In 2018, the median debt was $200,000.[17] And debt is associated with specialty choice—those with more debt are less likely to choose primary care, which pays less than other specialties.[18] Medicare already funds postgraduate medical education through residencies and fellowships. It's plausible that under M4A, Medicare could also subsidize or fully fund the cost of medical school and help pay down medical student debt. Though this would be a sizable cost, it would represent a very small proportion of the overall cost of M4A. Fully funding the cost of medical education could also help broaden the medical workforce, potentially attracting a more diverse pool of applicants given deep disparities in medical student debt by race. Indeed, one survey found that Black medical students were 19 percent more likely to graduate with more than $150,000 in debt than their white counterparts.[19]

LABOR

Historically, the American labor movement has had a complicated relationship with national health insurance. As discussed in Chapter 2, labor unions were largely opposed to the compulsory health insurance plans during the Progressive Era in the 1910s but emerged as one of the most powerful supporters of Medicare in the 1960s. Labor's historical ambivalence has also marked the early stages of the M4A debate.

Some labor groups have been skeptical of single-payer healthcare because they feel that many unions have already been able to win their members good health benefits, even at the expense of concessions on wages. But many labor groups see this as a powerful argument *for* single-payer: because negotiations over healthcare take up such a large proportion of collective bargaining efforts, separating health insurance from employment would free up space to negotiate a broader suite of benefits and focus on wage increases. In the words of union president Sara Nelson, "What we legislate, we don't have to negotiate."[20] The United Auto Workers strike against General Motors (GM) in 2019 offers a helpful case study. One of GM's first responses to the strike was to cut off worker health insurance support, leaving their striking workers without the healthcare they had once bargained for.[21] It illustrates the precariousness of employer-provided insurance, and these experiences may drive increasing union support for M4A.

Crucially, union support for M4A is stronger today than it has been in many prior pushes for national health insurance. This is largely owing to the efforts that congressional leaders and M4A organizers have put in to bring labor to the table early in the process, plus the fact that union health insurance has faced escalating cost pressures similar to other job-based insurance. Indeed, M4A has racked up an impressive list of endorsements from labor organizations, including some of the largest unions in the country: for instance, United Auto Workers, National Education Association, International Association of Machinists and Aerospace Workers, American Federation of Government Employees, American Postal Workers Union, and Amalgamated Transit Union, in addition to healthcare unions like National Nurses United and Service Employees International Union (discussed in Chapter 8).[22] According to a statement from NNU, "Unions representing a majority of union workers in the United States—over 9 million workers—have endorsed these bills. . . . We are at historic levels of labor support for this legislation, a fact of which we are extremely proud."[23]

A key policy provision for unions would be the opportunity to renegotiate their benefits if M4A passes, so that benefits won during collective bargaining would not simply be vacated without transferring them into other means of compensation. Toward this end, and in response to pressure from labor unions, Senator Sanders added a stipulation by which unions would be able to renegotiate contracts under the supervision of the National Labor Relations Board if M4A were to be implemented.[24] Similarly, Senator Warren's plan for M4A would have allowed employers to reduce their Medicare contribution if they passed the savings on to union workers in the form of increased wages, pensions, or other benefits achieved through collective bargaining.[25]

SENIORS

The clear concern for seniors is the sustainability of Medicare as we know it. Medicare today faces a simple challenge: Americans are aging. Every day, more Americans become eligible for Medicare, but the population of working-age Americans paying into the system has not kept pace. Consequently, the financial sustainability of both Medicare and Social Security has become an issue of widening concern.

Prior to the 2018 midterm elections, *USA Today* published an op-ed by Donald Trump attacking M4A as a threat to the sustainability of Medicare. He wrote, "I also made a solemn promise to our great seniors to protect Medicare. That is why

I am fighting so hard against the Democrats' plan that would eviscerate Medicare. . . . Democrats would gut Medicare with their planned government takeover of American health care."[26] The logic here is as simple and attractive as it is broken. The logic argues that as more people rely on Medicare, the Medicare "pie" will be split over more people, reducing the resources available for people on the program already. But that's not how M4A would work: the Medicare pie itself would get far larger under M4A as younger Americans pay more into the system. And while Trump implies that seniors on Medicare today would subsidize care for everyone else under M4A, the exact opposite appears to be true: the new revenue under M4A would subsidize expanded benefits for seniors currently on the program.

Indeed, M4A would not gut the existing Medicare program; in fact, it would expand it. Medicare today has numerous shortcomings that M4A could remedy, and so the crucial policy question for seniors will be *what* Medicare would cover under M4A.

One of the pain points for seniors is the high and rapidly increasing cost of prescription drugs. Although only about 12 percent of Americans are over the age of sixty-five, they account for 30 percent of all prescription drug use.[27] Seniors on Medicare need to buy separate prescription drug coverage sold by private companies. If M4A provides a robust prescription drug benefit that provides drugs at low cost, it could be a key leverage point to earn support from seniors.

Long-term care also continues to be a serious challenge for older Americans. The average long-term care facility costs about $225 a night (nearly $7,000 a month).[28] Including a long-term care benefit for seniors in M4A (which current House and Senate bills incorporate) could be a critical way to ensure that the move to M4A provides seniors with palpably better coverage.

Medicare today also doesn't cover vision, hearing, and dental care. Indeed, among Medicare beneficiaries, estimates suggest that about 75 percent who needed hearing devices did not have them and 70 percent who had dental challenges did not go to a dentist in the past year.[29] Under current House and Senate M4A bills, all these types of care would be covered—and this could have a sizable impact on seniors' quality of life (and support for M4A).

Seniors on Medicare also face high out-of-pocket costs for hospital and physician care. In 2019 the average American senior citizen reported pulling out $3,789 in savings to cover healthcare costs.[30] For one in four seniors, medical costs consume more than 20 percent of total income.[31] Medicare also fails to set a cap on total out-of-pocket costs, leaving seniors with tenuous financial protection in the case of serious illness or injury. M4A supporters will seek to emphasize the significant out-of-pocket savings that M4A could deliver, and also the fact that seniors likely would not have to keep paying for supplemental Medigap plans to fill the holes in their coverage.

The bottom line is that M4A could offer far better coverage than the current Medicare program (with the details depending on the design of the legislation). The challenge will be to educate seniors on the financial protections and benefits covered by M4A, and to earn their trust that extending Medicare to others won't cause them harm.

A final difficulty is the fact that current M4A bills propose to eliminate Medicare Advantage plans, the privately operated managed care programs supported by Medicare. Just over a third of seniors are on Medicare Advantage. These plans cost the government more overall but are attractive to seniors who are willing to accept more restrictions on their care in exchange for a wider range of benefits and lower out-of-pocket costs. Although M4A plans would also offer a wide range of benefits and little to no out-of-pocket costs, many seniors on Medicare Advantage are likely to resist the elimination of these plans in the same way that younger Americans worry about losing their employer-provided insurance.

LARGE EMPLOYERS

Major employers outside of healthcare are also important stakeholders in the health reform debate, though they face a different set of incentives than corporations within the healthcare industry. Because they spend billions of dollars annually providing healthcare for employees, their chief concern is the cost of healthcare. For example, in 2004 the biggest spender on employee healthcare in the country was General Motors, one of the world's biggest automotive manufacturers. GM spent about $4.5 billion annually to cover over 1.2 million workers, retirees, and family members—more than it spent on steel.[32] When the Great Recession struck in 2007–8, retiree healthcare costs were among the main reasons GM faced bankruptcy—and would become one of the most costly and important terms of the restructuring plan GM negotiated prior to being bailed out by the federal government.

Because they are focused on the cost of insurance, the critical calculation large employers will make regarding M4A is their bottom line: how much they would have to pay in healthcare costs under the current system, and how much they might pay in additional taxes under M4A. Senator Bernie Sanders has outlined a payment scheme that would include a 7.5 percent income-based premium levied on employers.[33] This plan could bring substantial savings to large employers in sectors that employ predominantly lower- to middle-income employees. As an example, consider a worker earning $50,000 annually for a family of four. In 2019, an average employer paid $14,561 per year for this family's healthcare.[34] Under Sanders's financing scheme, the same employer would pay $3,750 for the same family—a dramatic reduction. However, while private insurance premiums do not scale with income, this 7.5 percent income-based premium would. Therefore, it is possible that for employers in industries employing high-earning workers—such as financial services—healthcare costs could increase under M4A.

Senator Warren's M4A proposal includes an "employer Medicare contribution" priced at 98 percent of the average per-employee cost of healthcare prior to M4A, which experts estimate would save employers a collective $200 billion annually.[35]

Furthermore, large employers are currently exposed to rapidly increasing prices in the private healthcare market, whereas M4A could both get prices under control and give employers more stability regarding their annual healthcare costs. Businesses also spend a lot of money simply managing health benefits through human resources departments, and M4A would eliminate this bureaucratic expense.

The bottom line: if many (or even most) large employers would pay less for healthcare under M4A than they do today, that would be a powerful incentive for them to get behind the policy.

But healthcare is complicated. Beyond the dollars and cents, there are other reasons large employers might be reticent to support M4A. First, the current system offers large employers a competitive advantage over smaller businesses that could be erased under M4A. A large company today has the option to set up an insurance plan only for its own employees; these plans are subject to fewer regulations and taxes, and they can be particularly advantageous if a big company has an employee population that's healthier than the rest of the market. Partly as a result of this advantage, big companies can generally offer better insurance for every dollar spent: for instance, large and small employers paid about the same insurance premiums in 2019, but large businesses offered insurance with significantly lower deductibles.[36]

Some of America's largest corporations are making big investments in these in-house health plans. For example, Berkshire Hathaway, Amazon, and JPMorgan Chase, three of America's largest companies, teamed up to launch a new company called Haven Healthcare that will offer specially designed plans to employees and is expected to take an even more active role in managing its employees' healthcare. (The joint venture recruited celebrity physician Dr. Atul Gawande as its first CEO.) Similarly, Apple has launched its own primary care clinics for employees.[37] These in-house healthcare programs serve as yet another carrot to would-be employees. If large corporations begin to adopt this trend, massive upfront capital investments in these programs could serve as a direct disincentive for supporting M4A.

Ostensibly, under M4A large employers would want to continue to leverage benefits packages to attract talent. Therefore, one policy consideration that could sway support is whether or not employers could provide alternative types of insurance, and what coverage these alternatives could provide. In their current form, both the House and Senate M4A bills prohibit private insurance (including employee benefits) that duplicates the comprehensive services offered by M4A. However, employers would still be able to offer supplemental insurance or additional benefits such as concierge services that could, for example, advise employees about doctors to see, or handle booking appointments, transportation, and other logistics. It's also plausible that under M4A large employers could shift their benefits provisions to sustain their competitive advantage—improving family leave, childcare, vacation time, on-campus food and beverages, gym memberships, or other amenities.

M4A proponents will also need to contend with the ideological tilt of corporate leaders, who tend to be strongly suspicious of government involvement and taxation even if on paper they should save money under M4A. For instance, the US Chamber of Commerce—which, despite the official-sounding name, is a pro-business lobbying group that's been called "the premier voice for corporate power in Washington"—has adamantly opposed M4A and Medicare buy-in proposals.[38] (The US Chamber of Commerce is the largest single lobbying organization in the country, ranking even above PhRMA; it spent nearly $80 million on lobbying in 2019.)[39]

Still, for large companies whose political ideology does not prevent them from supporting M4A, the prospect of saving on healthcare costs could be powerful. These large employers are likely the only potential M4A allies with the financial resources to provide a counterweight to healthcare corporations in terms of expenditures on political campaign contributions, lobbying, and political advertising.

SMALL BUSINESSES

Small businesses have often sided politically with local and state chambers of commerce against government engagement and regulation. And chambers of commerce are often heavily influenced by local healthcare corporations. Nevertheless, providing healthcare to employees presents a major cost to small and midsized businesses, which lack the economies of scale of their larger counterparts. And as discussed earlier, smaller outfits often miss out on top talent because they cannot compete with the benefits packages offered by larger companies. Because of these dynamics (and their lower resources in general), small businesses often struggle to provide healthcare to their employees. Indeed, a nationwide poll of small business owners who offer healthcare benefits found that the "cost of providing healthcare coverage to employees" was most often cited as the biggest challenge they faced.[40] Many small businesses don't provide healthcare at all, making it difficult to attract and retain employees.

Representative Jayapal notes the support for M4A among small business owners: "I have had a lot of small business owners, including Republican small business owners, come up to me and say, 'You know what, I don't support anything else you stand for, but can you please pass Medicare for All?'"

For small businesses, the most important policy consideration that could sway support is the tax burden arising from M4A. Senator Sanders's payment scheme would omit taxes on the first $1 million in payroll, which means that many small businesses would pay nothing under this tax (most small businesses earn less than $1 million in revenue annually, including solo outfits where the owner is the only employee).[41] Similarly, under the Warren M4A proposal companies with fewer than fifty employees that are not paying for employee healthcare today would not need to pay into M4A. Whether defined in terms of payroll or number of employees, the level of this tax floor could have important implications for small business support—the higher the floor goes, the greater the number (and the larger the size) of businesses that would be exempted, increasing small business support.

Though small businesses lack the same financial heft as their larger counterparts, they do employ nearly half of the American workforce, and they maintain a level of trust with local communities that larger corporations often lack.[42] They are a trusted arbiter about the larger economic impact of healthcare and the effects of M4A. In that respect, a grassroots coalition of small business leaders who support the policy have formed Business Leaders for Health Care Transformation (formerly known as Business for Medicare for All), an organization that advocates on behalf of "business owners who believe our health insurance costs should not increase every year by double digits."[43]

10
ORGANIZING VS. ADVERTISING

Having considered the views of the American people toward M4A, where critical healthcare stakeholders stand, and how money, trust, and people power are being deployed on either side, we turn our attention to how all of these forces come together in the M4A debate.

American history is filled with steady support for national health insurance, punctuated by periods of rising public support and intense political interest. However, these surges are quickly met by a clear counterforce from the opponents of health reform. To appreciate these dynamics, consider the last major effort for healthcare reform: the Affordable Care Act, which passed on a party-line vote. This was possible because Democrats controlled both houses of Congress in the two years following President Obama's historic election in 2008. The kind of political surges that allow for the passage of major legislation like the ACA are often transient, cresting in the critical first two years of a new presidency before time in office and the inevitable erosion of national political fray wear the administration down. Democrats seized on this window of opportunity to pass the most sweeping health reform since Medicare.

But even successful health reform can provoke bitter opposition. Indeed, the ACA reform was not kind to Democratic incumbents in swing districts. After the ACA passed, the 2010 midterms netted Republicans sixty-three seats in the House and six seats in the Senate, giving Republicans majorities in both chambers. Democrats in swing districts today may fear that any major health reform effort, even if successful, could cost them their political careers.

And that's in the circumstance where reform actually passes. The more common outcome for major health reform efforts is failure. Support for some form of universal healthcare was high leading up to every major healthcare debate in American history—whether Franklin Roosevelt's abandoned reform during the New Deal, Truman's proposed overhaul in the 1940s, the Kennedy-Johnson push for Medicare in the 1960s, the Nixon health insurance plan, the Clinton-era overhaul, or the Obama debates.[1] However, most of these efforts failed completely. Politicians are not eager to stake their careers on a risky legislative push.

Much of that failure can be explained by targeted opposition from powerful, extremely wealthy interest groups, which ramp up their efforts to sway public opinion just as reform begins to look politically possible. This happens in two ways. Paid advertising aims to shape public opinion directly. But the indirect, secondary impact is to change the conversation we are having about healthcare—whether between individuals at a hair salon or in the "earned media," where journalists and pundits put health reform on public display. In our current debate, opponents seek to reframe that conversation away from the merits of M4A and toward the attacks against it: that M4A would take away your private insurance, raise your taxes, let the government control your healthcare, and take away jobs. Over the years powerful organizations have targeted the American public through political spending in the form of massive media campaigns that shift the national conversation and sour the public mood as important negotiations take place—think of the Campaigns, Inc. opposition to Truman's reforms, or the Harry and Louise ads of the 1990s. The threat of unleashing these destructive campaigns gives the wealthy opponents of health reform impressive influence over Congress, and they are experts at exploiting the veto points in our political system to erect a wall around the status quo.

How can these obstacles be overcome?

WHAT IT WILL TAKE FOR CONGRESS TO PASS MEDICARE FOR ALL

If history is any guide, a serious push for M4A will require electing a president who makes M4A a significant piece of her platform. But even if and when voters elect a pro-M4A president, passing a Medicare for All bill will require a supportive Congress.

We live in an era of tremendous political polarization. Given the clear opposition to M4A among today's elected Republicans, the bare minimum to make M4A possible is unified Democratic control of the White House and both chambers of Congress. Bipartisan health reform is a laudable goal, but remember that the Affordable Care Act—which was based on a plan implemented by a Republican governor and which hinged on giving tax credits to buy private insurance—gained not a single Republican vote. For the foreseeable future, it appears that any significant expansion of health coverage either will be a partisan effort or will not happen at all.

Of course, securing Democratic majorities is just step one. Within Congress, M4A will face several major barriers.

One barrier is the Senate filibuster, which can be used to block legislation that garners less than sixty votes. For M4A to have a chance in the Senate, Democrats need to either control sixty seats or circumvent the filibuster. There is a broader political debate about the merits of repealing the filibuster altogether, given that it can leave our legislature in almost perpetual gridlock no matter whom the people elect to represent them. There is also an existing process called reconciliation where legislation impacting the federal budget is immune to the filibuster (indeed, it was used to help pass the Affordable Care Act). Experts disagree on how much of M4A would be eligible for reconciliation, but taking this route would certainly present difficulties.

That still leaves the more foundational challenge: garnering enough congressional supporters to form a majority in favor of M4A. Democrats support many health reform ideas. A Democratic Congress will consider not just M4A but potentially the full suite of reform plans discussed in Chapter 6. One challenge here is that as of 2019–20, many members of Congress who support M4A also support alternative bills to expand Medicare; likewise, most voters who support M4A also support a public option.[2] Furthermore, early congressional debates will take place in committees responsible for healthcare legislation (like the Ways and Means Committee, which blocked Medicare during JFK's presidency); these are usually chaired by senior legislators, who may be more moderate than a new crop of Democrats elected to form a majority.

As Democrats debate which reform path to pursue, members of Congress from swing districts will protest that supporting M4A will cost them their next election—as it did for many Democrats who voted for the ACA. Congressional leadership often places enormous importance on keeping the party majority together in future elections; after all, majority control is critical not just for healthcare but also for all of the party's other domestic and international priorities. For that reason, congressional leaders give special weight to the concerns of moderate members facing difficult elections, taking for granted that deep-blue districts will continue sending Democrats to Congress.

When a serious congressional debate about M4A does begin, legislators will quickly confront the policy choices detailed in Chapter 4. Hospitals and physicians will argue that proposed payment rates are too low. Insurance companies will argue that Medicare Advantage for All is a better way forward. Pharmaceutical companies will warn that allowing the government to negotiate drug prices will destroy the incentive to make innovative medications. Funding for abortion and coverage for undocumented immigrants will become political flash points.

In debating these policy choices, legislators will also be mindful of the overall cost of the bill, knowing that the Congressional Budget Office will release an official cost estimate for any serious proposal. Legislators concerned about cost might consider whether to design a Medicare for All program that puts more out-of-pocket costs on patients or includes a less comprehensive benefit package. Legislators will also need to build support for a plan to finance M4A, knowing that any proposal to shift the heaviest burden of healthcare costs off the poor and middle class and onto the wealthy and corporations will face opposition from the latter two groups.

One further note. Alternative proposals to expand public health insurance—whether it's called a public option, Medicare buy-in, Medicare for America, or something else—will face most of these same barriers. They will be opposed by Republicans in Congress. They will be opposed by pharmaceutical companies, insurance companies, and many hospitals. They will face the inevitable snags of legislative debate, will need to navigate political flash points, and must weather being smeared as "socialism" and "a government takeover of healthcare."

It is not possible to avoid these barriers. The question is what it will take to overcome them. Ultimately, what will be needed is strong political will within the Democratic Party to pursue M4A. Though passage will not require unanimous Democratic support, M4A will need to become a high priority for Democratic voters and their representatives, and popular enough in swing districts to support Democratic legislators who endorse it. This new consensus is necessary to bolster support among legislators who face the possibility of losing their seats if it passes.

What would it take to strengthen the consensus on M4A and build the political will for reform? There is only one foreseeable possibility: a popular national movement pushing for M4A. Quite simply, there is no other force strong enough to overcome the partisan attacks and the deep-pocketed opposition from industry.

Make no mistake: a public option or Medicare buy-in would need a similar popular movement to overcome partisan and corporate opposition. In fact, the only reform packages that likely wouldn't have to rely on broad public support are incremental reforms that hinge on winning over moderate Republicans or the healthcare industry.

That was the strategy of the Affordable Care Act; although hopes of bipartisanship were ultimately futile, efforts to win over the healthcare industry largely succeeded. But that strategy is not available for a public option or Medicare buy-in because elected Republicans and healthcare industry groups oppose those proposals as well, deliberately lumping them together with M4A and using the same attack lines. (Exhibit A from the Big Healthcare opposition group: "Medicare for All, Medicare Buy-In, and a public option all mean the same thing: you'd pay more to wait longer for worse care.")[3]

This is one area where M4A has a political advantage over more incremental reforms as a policy to organize around. M4A is a simple policy that expresses a clear moral value: healthcare is a human right. And it has the potential to deliver truly life-changing benefits to millions of Americans. Despite its other political vulnerabilities, there is no doubt that M4A has the potential to excite a broad swath of the American public.

We are already seeing this dynamic play out. In early 2020, Melinda St. Louis of the advocacy group Public Citizen told us, "The grassroots constituency, and the movement, is all Medicare for All. You don't hear a movement for a public option." If *any* universal healthcare plan is to pass in Congress, the linchpin of its success will be a grassroots constituency that builds popular support for the policy and harnesses the excitement of supporters into an organized movement to drive the political process toward reform. Whether M4A or a public option, success or failure will depend critically on the strength of the movement behind it.

The COVID-19 pandemic offers that movement tremendous tailwinds by showing just how ill-prepared our healthcare system was to cope with the country's worst health crisis in three generations. As it devastated American lives and livelihoods, the coronavirus revealed the precariousness of American healthcare. COVID-19 nearly overwhelmed our healthcare system, which struggled to provide basic resources to patients and providers at the scale needed to face the pandemic—all while the accompanying economic downturn left millions of people without health insurance.

Translating this frustration with the state of American healthcare into political action will require thoughtful, goal-directed organizing. Let's dive into the role of organizing in pushing M4A, and then look at how deep-pocketed opponents will fight back with advertising to try to undo that progress.

ORGANIZING

Lacking the power and resources of major corporations, the forces for M4A will leverage their organizing power to shape public opinion. In fact, when it comes to shaping lasting changes in popular support, organizing may actually be more powerful than political connections or financial resources. To appreciate the power of organizing to shape our perspectives on an issue, consider the change in public attitudes toward same-sex marriage. The Pew Research Center has been tracking attitudes on same-sex marriage in America since the early 2000s.[4] In 2004, 60 percent of Americans opposed same-sex marriage, and only 31 percent supported it. But by 2017, 62 percent of Americans supported it, and only 32 percent opposed it. What happened? People organized to change hearts and minds. Once those changes came about, the laws followed. In his book *Engines of Liberty: The Power of Citizen Activists to Make Constitutional Law*, lead ACLU attorney David Cole details how movements of ordinary people organized to shape public opinion on same-sex marriage, well before Massachusetts legalized it and the Supreme Court ruled same-sex marriage bans unconstitutional. He writes that the Supreme Court decision "is unimaginable absent the decades of advocacy of small groups of committed individuals."[5]

There are further parallels as well. The movement for same-sex marriage rested on a basic moral argument that could be expressed clearly (e.g., "Love is love"), and people from many walks of life were familiar with the struggles faced by same-sex couples. The movement for M4A contains similar features, with a clear moral argument (e.g., "Healthcare is a human right") and struggles with the US healthcare system cutting across traditional divides. (Absent in the same-sex marriage debates, of course, was a $4 trillion industry whose profits were threatened by reform.)

The rise of the internet has supercharged movement organizing. In his book *We've Got People: From Jesse Jackson to Alexandria Ocasio-Cortez, the End of Big Money and the*

Rise of a Movement, journalist Ryan Grim details how the internet has enabled public advocacy organizations and progressive political campaigns to connect, organize people, and raise money in innovative ways.[6] Targeted social media and email campaigns allow these organizations to raise millions in small amounts, relying on $5 or $10 contributions from many small donors rather than $5,000 or $10,000 checks from a select group of wealthy individuals or big corporations. But rather than spend these millions on advertising campaigns, they spend on organizing, building grassroots people power. They use tactics like door-to-door canvassing to take a message to people's homes, where they find new supporters to join the movement. They use civil disobedience and "bird-dogging"—putting politicians on the spot in public or on camera to answer for their political opinions—to earn media attention, convey a sense of moral urgency, and reframe the public conversation about the merits of an idea.

Consider the opposition to the ACA repeal efforts in the first two years of the Trump presidency. Grassroots organizations such as the Center for Popular Democracy, Public Citizen, MoveOn, and the Women's March made opposing ACA repeal a major goal of their efforts. They coordinated massive canvasses across the country, focusing on swing districts and vulnerable legislators such as Senators Jeff Flake (R-AZ) and Susan Collins (R-ME). They bird-dogged politicians to create viral moments on social media and conducted massive sit-ins in the halls of Congress. Their efforts attracted tremendous support on social media and garnered headlines, their earned media coverage counteracting the paid commercials of their opposition. Leaders such as Ady Barkan, a progressive organizer diagnosed with ALS in 2016, emerged as key voices in these fights, both illuminating the human stakes of ACA repeal and embodying the spirit of the organizing efforts to oppose it. Though ACA repeal was thought to be inevitable, the organizers ultimately won.

It is often said that fighting *against* a policy—like ACA repeal—is easier than fighting *for* a policy. But grassroots organizing has also been used to successfully fight for Medicaid expansion in red states through citizen-initiated ballot initiatives. In 2018, for instance, led by a grassroots movement known as Reclaim Idaho, the Medicaid ballot initiative in Idaho passed with 61 percent of the vote—in a state where 60 percent of voters supported Donald Trump two years earlier.[7]

Grassroots organizing will be critical to passing M4A in two ways. First and most obviously, it will be critical in driving consensus on the policy among the public. At its best, organizing puts the message in the mouth of the most trusted informant of all, the public itself. It empowers people to commune around the ideals of the world they want to live in together. Rather than utilizing a glitzy thirty-second commercial featuring actors portraying your next-door neighbor, strong organizing means that the person reaching out to you is *actually* your next-door neighbor. By putting power into the hands of the people who are most affected by a policy, organizing amplifies the significance of that policy all the more.

Alongside these efforts, grassroots organizing will be critical in electing representatives who believe in the policy. In many respects, this is already happening. Democrats are moving left.[8] One telling indicator here is people's response to the statement "Government should do more to help the needy." In 1994, 58 percent of Democrats agreed, while 38 percent of Republicans did. In 2017, 71 percent of Democrats agreed, compared to 24 percent of Republicans.[9]

Because the positions of politicians are more directly shaped by the opinions and beliefs of the most vocal members of their parties, it is likely that leftward movement among the activist base has contributed to more left-leaning positions for Democratic candidates—including support for M4A. Organizations such as Justice Democrats and Our Revolution have sprung up with the express intent of supporting progressive challengers in safe Democratic seats. For them, M4A has emerged as an important political litmus test within the Democratic Party.

A key step in that evolution was Senator Bernie Sanders's 2016 primary campaign for president, when he made M4A a cornerstone issue on his platform. Positioning himself in a heated primary to the left of Secretary Hillary Clinton for the Democratic nomination, he was able to set up his support of M4A as an implicit contrast with the Clintons' failed attempt at more complex reform in the 1990s. After the 2016 primary, M4A has remained a point of demarcation between more centrist and progressive Democrats. Clearly, the debate about M4A has been deeply influenced by—and deeply influences—America's changing conversation about its politics.

But it is also a sign of the power of organizing. Bernie Sanders's 2016 campaign was a watershed moment in demonstrating how grassroots political campaigns could be built, funded, and driven by big organizing. Rather than courting wealthy donors, Sanders raised hundreds of millions of dollars across hundreds of thousands of contributors, famously receiving an average of $27 a donation. He leveraged a "distributed" organizing model, empowering volunteers with the digital tools to organize independently, rather than organizing the campaign from the top down.

That approach to organizing spurred a raft of progressive primary challengers for Congress, Senate, and governorships in 2018 and 2020. Using many of the same organizing and fundraising tactics that were pioneered by the Sanders campaign, new pro-M4A leaders like Alexandria Ocasio-Cortez (who were supported by groups like Justice Democrats) defeated more centrist incumbents who opposed the policy. To be sure, many progressive challengers who supported M4A did not win their elections, but organizers see these races as just the beginning of a much longer movement.

In heavily Democratic districts, it may only be a matter of time until the people elect representatives who share their views on M4A: from 2018 through 2020, between 75 percent and 80 percent of self-identified Democratic voters consistently supported M4A, according to polls by the Kaiser Family Foundation.[10]

In time, swing districts and states will emerge as the ultimate battlegrounds over M4A. Will M4A appeal to moderate Democrats, independents, and even moderate Republicans? Polls showing majority support from independents give M4A proponents cause for cautious optimism, but the proof will be in the election outcomes. More to the point, acceptance of M4A by moderate Democratic voters and independents is one of the central goals of organizing on this issue, bringing M4A fully into the mainstream through education and advocacy.

Big organizing is already changing the tenor of Congress in favor of M4A. The victories of progressive challengers have a knock-on impact on Democratic incumbents, signaling that failing to support progressive policies like M4A may make them a target for challengers who will. Indeed, after 2018 a number of previously uncommitted members of Congress came out in support of the policy. This is a clear illustration of pitting people power against financial power. The corporate opposition tries to make legislators fear for their political careers if they support M4A, threatening well-funded advertising campaigns against them in their districts. Movement organizers make legislators fear their election prospects if they *oppose* M4A. The leverage of organizers is not money, but the ability to drive constituents to town halls and campaign rallies demanding support for M4A—plus a willingness to run primary challenges against them if other efforts are insufficient.

This organizing approach to passing M4A is baked into the construction of the actual legislation. Representative Pramila Jayapal brought movement leaders to the table to help design the M4A bill, recognizing that their support would be critical to passing it. "The challenge of hundreds of millions of dollars spent by insurance companies and drug companies to beat this back can only be overcome by a massive groundswell of people across the country," she told us. "We were aware of that when writing it, we were aware of that introducing it. And we're still aware of that as we continue to try to build momentum for the bill on the outside and we push for more people to come in on the inside."

This political strategy is in stark contrast to the strategy used to pass the Affordable Care Act. The designers of the ACA brought the healthcare industry to the table early, cutting deals and writing the bill to win the support of pharmaceutical companies, the hospital industry, and insurance companies (though that last effort would prove unsuccessful). Leaders in the M4A effort are adopting a similar strategy, but the groups at the table look very different: they are nurses, labor leaders, and grassroots organizers. Both the architects of the ACA and the architects of M4A recognized the importance of building a coalition of supportive stakeholders. But the stakeholders in these two cases are very different, both in terms of their identities and in the nature of their power.

This is where the swing stakeholders discussed in Chapter 9 could be crucial. Doctors, unions, seniors, large employers, and small businesses could be critical partners to make a popular movement more effective. Physicians and business leaders are trusted community members who can help shape the public conversation and the tenor of media coverage. Large employers could supply some financial heft. Unions are critical hubs of people power. And all these groups have strong political relationships, which could help provide a counterweight to the industry opponents.

ADVERTISING

The opponents of M4A will seek to undermine public opinion and block political action using very different sources of power. We don't need to speculate about their strategy; it's already in motion.

At the center of the opposition to M4A is a group called the Partnership for America's Healthcare Future. Despite the public-spirited name, the Partnership is a coalition of more than a hundred healthcare industry groups and corporate trade associations, including America's Health Insurance Plans, Federation of American Hospitals, Pharmaceutical Research and Manufacturers of America, Blue Cross Blue Shield Association, and the Biotechnology Innovation Organization.[11] The Partnership expressed two initial objectives in documents leaked in November 2018:

1. Change the national conversation around single payer/ Medicare for All.

2. Minimize the potential for this option in healthcare from becoming part of a national political party's platform in 2020.[12]

The group received $5.1 million in the second half of 2018 alone. It was extremely active during the 2018 midterms and 2020 Democratic primaries, influencing Democratic talking points in several important races and downplaying the successes (and hyping up the failures) of candidates running on the Medicare for All platform. They spent $300,000 on digital media ads alone during the 2018 cycle and 2020 primary.[13] In the summer of 2019 they bought half of all political advertising in Iowa, then spent $1.2 million in advance of the Iowa caucuses in March 2020.[14] They bought millions of dollars more in advertising throughout the Democratic presidential primary season. One television ad aired during the Democratic debates features several actors portraying a diverse group of busy middle-class Americans going about their daily lives and speaking straight to the camera about healthcare. Says one: "We don't want to be forced into a one-size-fits-all government insurance system."[15]

The Partnership is already following a well-worn playbook: aggressive advertising spending that drives a lobbying machine focused on dissuading representatives in key districts from supporting reform.[16] Over the past two decades, the pharmaceutical, insurance, and hospital industries have spent nearly $9 billion in collective lobbying.[17] Through front groups like the Partnership, they stand to invest substantially more in this advertising-driven lobbying strategy. After all, these industries have a long history of defeating healthcare reform proposals using these tactics.

The opponents of health reform are extraordinarily savvy. They understand well the pitfalls that M4A will face in Congress, they know which legislators will be on the fence about supporting it, and they understand how to make those lawmakers fear for their political careers if they take the "wrong" position on M4A. These groups have enough money that virtually overnight they could fund an overwhelming campaign in a legislator's home district—through TV, radio, newspaper, and targeted social media ads—charging that Representative So-and-So is supporting a socialist takeover that will take away your healthcare and raise your taxes. Legislators also know that these corporations can contribute handsomely to any future opponents' election campaign. The Partnership can arrange to have the CEO of the local hospital—which might be the largest employer in that congressional district—meet with the representative to express her concerns that M4A will harm care for the entire community; the Partnership might even ghostwrite an op-ed for that CEO to publish under her name in the local paper. Industry opponents know that all of these efforts will help achieve their goal of changing the national conversation around health reform by changing the frame around earned media for M4A so that it's focused more on the attack lines rather than the merits.

For any legislator skittish about supporting M4A for fear it will hurt her election chances in her moderate hometown, the power of these tactics cannot be underestimated. These tactics also reveal a connection between corporate opposition to health reform and centrist Democratic opposition. For progressive Democrats who rely on a progressive base to get elected—perhaps from a deep-blue district—the scare tactics and media campaigns of the corporate opposition are less of a threat, because public support for M4A is firmer. (That's one reason groups like Justice Democrats put such a high priority on electing progressive Democrats in these safe deep-blue districts.) But for Democrats from swing districts who rely on a combination of progressives, moderates, and independents to win their elections, the threat of industry-funded attack campaigns is more severe because public support for M4A is more malleable. As a result, much of the battle for M4A will center on these swing voters and members of Congress who can either complete the M4A coalition or deny it.

Let's pause for a moment and zoom out. Having laid out the battle that will ensue between the big organizing of the M4A movement and the big money of its opponents, as well as the treacherous maze that awaits M4A in the legislature, it's worth asking a simple question: if most Americans support M4A, why is it so difficult to pass? Beyond opposition from those who profit from the status quo, a more complete answer requires us to confront the ways in which the views of the people do and do not get transmitted into American government.

First, in the weeks and months leading up to an election, public opinion can shift based on the messages and arguments to which voters are exposed. Because of the Supreme Court's 2010 decision in *Citizens United vs. Federal Election Commission*, corporations can spend unlimited sums of money seeking to influence elections—for instance, attacking candidates who support M4A, and propagating negative messages (and even misinformation) about the policy. This threatens public opinion before people even get a chance to make it to the polls. And because political campaigns are funded through private donations, candidates have a financial advantage if they adopt platforms that are favored by wealthy individuals and businesses. This advantage is bolstered by the unlimited spending that corporations can engage in to support or oppose candidates. All these forces make it more difficult for candidates who support policies like M4A to make it onto the ballot and win.

Even at the polls, voter suppression tactics make it more difficult for Americans to exercise their right to vote. As the American Civil Liberties Union explains it, "Since 2008, states across the country have passed measures to make it harder for Americans—particularly Black people, the elderly, students, and people with disabilities—to exercise their fundamental right to cast a ballot. These measures include cuts to early voting, voter ID laws, and purges of voter rolls."[18]

There are other barriers. Gerrymandering, where congressional maps are drawn to advantage one political party, means that a minority of voters in a state can often elect a majority of representatives. The Senate map misallocates voters as well: 40 million Americans living in California elect the same number of senators as the 570,000 Americans living in Wyoming—a 70-to-1 disparity. And the Electoral College means that a president can be seated even if more Americans voted for the other candidate.

Therefore, the movement for health reform—especially M4A, but virtually all other major reforms as well—shares common cause with the movement to strengthen our democracy more broadly. M4A is premised on the idea that government can take bold action to promote the general welfare. Reforms to our political institutions are of the same spirit, aiming to restore the people's faith in the government that the Constitution erected in their name.

SO, IS IT POSSIBLE?

M4A is possible. But it is not inevitable. If it happens, it will have been because the right policy choices attracted the right coalition, which used the right tactics to elect the right officials in the right moment for change.

The backbone of any push for M4A must be a popular national movement pressing for reform. There is no foreseeable path to M4A becoming law without this groundswell of people bolstering public opinion and exerting political pressure in the face of extraordinarily well-funded opposition.

A broadened coalition of stakeholders would also be an enormous boon. That coalition could include doctors who have had it with a labyrinthine healthcare system that fails patients on a daily basis—even if it means taking on the powerful hospitals that employ them. It might include businesses of all sizes who choose their own bottom line over the healthcare industry's. It might include labor unions who appreciate that securing healthcare as a guaranteed right will only strengthen their hand. It might include seniors who recognize that M4A expands Medicare rather than guts it. Finally, and perhaps most important, it will require all of them to band together with grassroots organizers against the fearmongering of healthcare corporations who will spend—and have already spent—millions to tell us that M4A is too expensive, is too unreliable, and will take away what little we already have.

The terrain might shift in other ways, too. Perhaps the battle of ideas will tilt toward M4A, swaying elite opinion and transforming the tenor of media coverage. Perhaps centrist Americans will start to view M4A not as an impractical and radical dream but as a serious proposal to deliver on the promise of universal healthcare while tackling America's unique cost drivers. Perhaps we will pass democratic reforms that make the views of Congress more representative of the American people's views. Perhaps we will change the very way that we think and talk about healthcare: we might think of physicians not so much as providers of a commodity but as caregivers and partners in healing; we might think of hospitals not so much as businesses but as community institutions; we might think of ourselves not so much as consumers but as patients and citizens.

M4A is not inevitable, but there's no doubt that the direction of change makes this outcome more probable. More Americans are finding healthcare unaffordable, inaccessible, and ineffective. The experience of giving and receiving healthcare has been corroded by a broken system that too often puts industry profits above the needs of the sick. All of this has left us with the most expensive healthcare system in the world, where tens of millions of Americans are priced out of care, and those who can get care are paying dearly for it. The corporations that profit from overpriced healthcare will continue to join their allies to spend on advertising campaigns, lobby elected officials, and perform small acts of charity in the name of good health to change public opinion in their favor. They have succeeded through these tactics in the past. And they are doing it again.

But if M4A happens, it will be because the American public decides that we can, in fact, have a more just, equitable, and sustainable system—that we can rise beyond the insecurity that says that the status quo is the best we can have, and choose to engage in the work of creating the system.

11

PARTING THOUGHTS

Throughout this book, we've sought to provide you with an honest, approachable assessment of Medicare for All—its opportunities and challenges, and its potential for the future.

M4A is single-payer healthcare that uses collective public action through government to provide universal health insurance across the United States, thereby vastly limiting the powers of the for-profit insurance industry, hospital industry, and pharmaceutical industry. Though it would require a massive government investment in healthcare, there's ample reason to believe M4A could cost the American people less overall by eliminating much of the bloated overhead needed to prop up our current system and by cracking down on the industry's ability to charge high prices for care. By trading insurance premiums for taxes and slashing out-of-pocket costs,

M4A has the potential to put more money into the pockets of most American families. Quite simply, most Americans could pay less for better, more secure health coverage.

There remain a number of important questions about how the policy would be designed. These include what goods and services M4A would cover, how it would pay for them, and what role would be left for private insurance. Questions also include how to transition to M4A, which will result in a massive workforce churn that will not be without consequence for hundreds of thousands of Americans currently employed in our healthcare system.

And the politics are treacherous. Passing M4A would require standing up to deeply entrenched private interests in order to launch a massive reinvestment in government public goods. In that respect, the public conversation about M4A may be about more than just healthcare.

We wrote this book because much of the public conversation has been marked by a general lack of engagement with what M4A really means, how it works, and what the challenges ahead actually are. The conversation has often devolved into a series of broad, sweeping claims about what the policy is and is not. However, the discussion about M4A is, in some ways, the opening salvo in a broader debate about the role of American government in solving big American problems.

Here some historical context may be helpful. Empowered by the idea of promoting "the general welfare," American government as we know it today emerged from a bipartisan consensus around the critical role of government in providing basic public goods that grew out of the Progressive Era in the 1910s and 1920s and took hold during the New Deal in the 1930s and 1940s. The idea that government could—and should—solve large-scale problems, including in public education, infrastructure, and even healthcare (to some degree), was a hallmark of this era. That approach to government wasn't limited to Democrats: the American highway system we take for granted today was built under the Eisenhower administration, and no Republican would dare repeal Social Security or Medicare.

During the Reagan era, however, a new bipartisan governing consensus emerged. It holds that in America the free market should provide goods and services, whether we're talking about a Rolls-Royce or basic healthcare. That era saw the introduction of private capital into previously public goods, like public education in the form of charter school programs, or public infrastructure in the form of privatization of airports and public transit systems. Though this movement was kicked off in the Reagan years by slashing taxes, public programs, and the infrastructure of government itself, the basic logic has persisted through subsequent administrations, both Republican and Democratic. Indeed, the primacy of the private market remained a hallmark of the presidencies of Bill Clinton—famous for his "Third Way"—and Barack Obama as well. Their healthcare plans reflected a complicated dance between government regulation and private insurance, but both proposed essentially market-driven solutions for healthcare reform.

However, the public consensus may be shifting again. The Great Recession exposed many Americans to a level of poverty and insecurity that hadn't been seen in America since the Great Depression—which the New Deal was originally created to solve. Rising inequality paralleling the Gilded Age has left a large swath of the country without stable, secure employment or basic access to healthcare. COVID-19 exposed tens of millions of Americans to the insecurity of the systems that the old governing consensus had wrought. More than 100,000 Americans died in just over 100 days of a pandemic that our public health system should have largely prevented. More than 20 million Americans lost jobs, kicking off what could become, as one economist called it, a "Greater Depression," and millions got kicked off of their health insurance as a result.[1]

Both before and after COVID-19, many Americans are asking how the market-based governing consensus can solve their most urgent problems—and whether or not it created them in the first place.

This is the sociopolitical context within which we are debating M4A today, and why the conversation about M4A may be broader than just healthcare. In fact, the future of M4A may hinge instead on three far bigger questions:

1. Whether government should shoulder one of the largest and fastest-growing expenditures currently burdening American families
2. How best to provide a necessary good to all people equitably

3. Whether or not we believe in collective action in an increasingly diverse America

That third question is particularly poignant. It's likely that 2016 will be remembered most for the political earthquake of Donald Trump's election to the White House. However, perhaps the more important seismic shift that took place that year is that, for the first time in American history, the majority of newborn Americans were infants of color. The two changes are not unrelated. Indeed, many argue that Trump's election was a tribal response by low-income rural white voters to a changing American demographic, typified by the president he replaced. If that is true, it may not bode well for a collective approach to solving one of America's deepest collective problems, as tribal fault lines that shaped the Trump victory would abrogate any effort toward collective will.

Trump's election has alternatively been explained as a collective rebuke of the American political establishment, which has perpetuated the Reagan-era governing consensus on both sides of the aisle. In that explanation, a broad reinvestment in public goods, like M4A, is far more likely. Perhaps more than any other single policy, M4A would signify a decisive break with the past forty years of our politics and herald a new consensus about the society Americans aspire to live in.

Either way, the urgent problem of providing accessible, affordable, dependable, and equitable healthcare to Americans at scale remains. As we hope we've demonstrated, M4A is a viable solution to that problem.

NOTES

Introduction

1. Frank Whelan, "In the America of 1787, Big Families Are the Norm and Life Expectancy Is 38," *Morning Call*, June 28, 1987, https://www.mcall.com/news/mc-xpm-1987-06-28-2569915-story.html.
2. Kathryn MacKay, "Statistics on Slavery," Weber State University, https://faculty.weber.edu/kmackay/statistics_on_slavery.htm, accessed March 4, 2020.
3. Elizabeth Arias, "National Center for Health Statistics Data Brief No. 244," Centers for Disease Control and Prevention, 2016, https://www.cdc.gov/nchs/products/databriefs/db244.htm.
4. Max Roser, Hannah Ritchie, and Bernadeta Dadonaite, "Child and Infant Mortality," Our World in Data, November 2019, https://ourworldindata.org/child-mortality#child-mortality-around-the-world-since-1800.
5. Act for the Relief of Sick and Disabled Seamen (1798), https://history.nih.gov/research/downloads/1StatL605.pdf.
6. "Life Expectancy Increases in 2018 as Overdose Deaths Decline Along with Several Leading Causes of Death," CDC National Center for Health Statistics, January 30, 2020, https://www.cdc.gov/nchs/pressroom/nchs_press_releases/2020/202001_Mortality.htm.
7. Andrea M. Sisko et al., "National Health Expenditure Projections, 2018–27: Economic and Demographic Trends Drive Spending and Enrollment Growth," *Health Affairs* 38, no. 3 (February 20, 2019): 491–501, https://doi.org/10.1377/hlthaff.2018.05499; Centers for Medicare and Medicaid Services, "NHE Projections 2018–2027," https://www.cms.gov/Research-Statistics-Data-and-Systems/Statistics-Trends-and-Reports/NationalHealthExpendData/NationalHealthAccountsProjected, accessed March 4, 2020.
8. Adrienne M. Gilligan et al., "Death or Debt? National Estimates of Financial Toxicity in Persons with Newly-Diagnosed Cancer," *American Journal of Medicine* 131, no. 10 (2018), https://doi.org/10.1016/j.amjmed.2018.05.020.
9. John Nichols, "Health Care Through FDR's Lenses," NPR, March 22, 2010, https://www.npr.org/templates/story/story.

php?storyId=125007071; Teresa Ghilarducci, "Republicans' Public Opposition to Social Security and Medicare," *Forbes*, accessed March 4, 2020, https://www.forbes.com/sites/teresaghilarducci/2018/11/02/republican-public-opposition-to-social-security-and-medicare.

Chapter 1

1. Irene Papanicolas, Liana R. Woskie, and Ashish K. Jha, "Health Care Spending in the United States and Other High-Income Countries," *JAMA* 319, no. 10 (2018): 1024–39, https://doi.org/10.1001/jama.2018.1150.
2. Andrea M. Sisko et al., "National Health Expenditure Projections, 2018–27: Economic and Demographic Trends Drive Spending and Enrollment Growth," *Health Affairs* 38, no. 3 (February 20, 2019): 491–501, https://doi.org/10.1377/hlthaff.2018.05499.
3. National Center for Health Statistics, "Health, United States, 2015: With Special Feature on Racial and Ethnic Health Disparities," 2016, https://www.cdc.gov/nchs/data/hus/hus15.pdf.
4. Papanicolas, Woskie, and Jha, "Health Care Spending in the United States and Other High-Income Countries."
5. National Center for Health Statistics, "Health Insurance Coverage: Early Release of Estimates From the National Health Interview Survey, January-June 2019," 2019.
6. Papanicolas, Woskie, and Jha, "Health Care Spending in the United States and Other High-Income Countries."
7. National Center for Coverage Innovation at Families USA, "The COVID-19 Pandemic and Resulting Economic Crash Have Caused the Greatest Health Insurance Losses in American History," July 17, 2020, https://familiesusa.org/wp-content/uploads/2020/07/COV-254_Coverage-Loss_Report_7-17-20.pdf.
8. Centers for Medicare and Medicaid Services, "National Health Expenditure Accounts 2018," https://www.cms.gov/Research-Statistics-Data-and-Systems/Statistics-Trends-and-Reports/NationalHealthExpendData/NationalHealthAccountsHistorical, accessed March 4, 2020.
9. Sisko et al., "National Health Expenditure Projections, 2018–27"; Centers for Medicare and Medicaid Services, "NHE Projections 2018–2027," https://www.cms.gov/Research-Statistics-Data-and-Systems/Statistics-Trends-and-Reports/NationalHealthExpendData/NationalHealthAccountsProjected, accessed March 4, 2020.

10. Papanicolas, Woskie, and Jha, "Health Care Spending in the United States and Other High-Income Countries."
11. Rabah Kamal and Cynthia Cox, "How Do Healthcare Prices and Use in the U.S. Compare to Other Countries?," Peterson-KFF Health System Tracker, May 8, 2018, https://www.healthsystemtracker.org/chart-collection/how-do-healthcare-prices-and-use-in-the-u-s-compare-to-other-countries.
12. John Hargraves and Aaron Bloschichak, "International Comparisons of Health Care Prices from the 2017 IFHP Survey," Health Care Cost Institute, December 17, 2019, https://healthcostinstitute.org/hcci-research/international-comparisons-of-health-care-prices-2017-ifhp-survey.
13. Hargraves and Bloschichak, "International Comparisons of Health Care Prices from the 2017 IFHP Survey."
14. Gerard F. Anderson et al., "It's the Prices, Stupid: Why the United States Is So Different from Other Countries," *Health Affairs* 22, no. 3 (May 2003): 89–105, https://doi.org/10.1377/hlthaff.22.3.89.
15. Medicare.gov Procedure Price Lookup, "MRI Scan of Brain Before and After Contrast," 2020, https://www.medicare.gov/procedure-price-lookup/cost/70553.
16. Chapin White and Christopher Whaley, "Prices Paid to Hospitals by Private Health Plans Are High Relative to Medicare and Vary Widely: Findings from an Employer-Led Transparency Initiative," RAND Corporation, 2019, https://doi.org/10.7249/RR3033.
17. Insurance Information Institute, "Facts + Statistics: Insurance Industry Overview," 2019, https://www.iii.org/fact-statistic/facts-statistics-industry-overview.
18. Zack Cooper et al., "Variation in Health Spending Growth for the Privately Insured from 2007 to 2014," *Health Affairs* 38, no. 2 (February 1, 2019): 230–36, https://doi.org/10.1377/hlthaff.2018.05245.
19. Kaiser Family Foundation, "Premiums and Worker Contributions Among Workers Covered by Employer-Sponsored Coverage, 1999–2019," September 25, 2019, https://www.kff.org/interactive/premiums-and-worker-contributions-among-workers-covered-by-employer-sponsored-coverage-1999-2019.
20. Kaiser Family Foundation, "Employer Health Benefits: 2014 Annual Survey," 2014, http://files.kff.org/attachment/2014-employer-health-benefits-survey-full-report.

21. Brent D. Fulton, "Health Care Market Concentration Trends in the United States: Evidence and Policy Responses," *Health Affairs* 36, no. 9 (September 2017): 1530–38, https://doi.org/10.1377/hlthaff.2017.0556.
22. Kaufman Hall, "2017 in Review: The Year M&A Shook the Healthcare Landscape," 2018, https://www.kaufmanhall.com/ideas-resources/research-report/2017-review-year-ma-shook-healthcare-landscape.
23. Martin Gaynor and Robert Town, "The Impact of Hospital Consolidation—Update," Synthesis Project, Robert Wood Johnson Foundation, 2012, https://www.rwjf.org/content/dam/farm/reports/issue_briefs/2012/rwjf73261.
24. Margot Sanger-Katz, "The New Goliaths," *National Journal*, February 18, 2012.
25. Gaynor and Town, "The Impact of Hospital Consolidation—Update."
26. Michael R. McKellar et al., "Insurer Market Structure and Variation in Commercial Health Care Spending," *Health Services Research* 49, no. 3 (June 2014): 878–92, https://doi.org/10.1111/1475-6773.12131.
27. Glenn A. Melnick, Yu-Chu Shen, and Vivian Yaling Wu, "The Increased Concentration of Health Plan Markets Can Benefit Consumers Through Lower Hospital Prices," *Health Affairs* 30, no. 9 (September 2011): 1728–33, https://doi.org/10.1377/hlthaff.2010.0406.
28. Leemore Dafny, Mark Duggan, and Subramaniam Ramanarayanan, "Paying a Premium on Your Premium? Consolidation in the US Health Insurance Industry," *American Economic Review* 102, no. 2 (April 2012): 1161–85, https://doi.org/10.1257/aer.102.2.1161.
29. Complaint, *U.S. and State of Michigan v. Blue Cross Blue Shield of Michigan* (E.D. Mich., October 18, 2010), https://www.justice.gov/atr/case-document/complaint-43.
30. Steve Cicala, Ethan M. J. Lieber, and Victoria Marone, "Regulating Markups in US Health Insurance," *American Economic Journal: Applied Economics* 11, no. 4 (2019): 71–104.
31. Andrew Pollack, "Drug Goes from $13.50 a Tablet to $750, Overnight," *New York Times*, September 20, 2015, https://www.nytimes.com/2015/09/21/business/a-huge-overnight-increase-in-a-drugs-price-raises-protests.html.

32. Chris Woodyard and Mary Jo Layton, "Massive Price Increases on EpiPens Raise Alarm," *USA Today*, August 22, 2016, https://www.usatoday.com/story/money/business/2016/08/22/two-senators-urge-scrutiny-epipen-price-boost/89129620.
33. Papanicolas, Woskie, and Jha, "Health Care Spending in the United States and Other High-Income Countries."
34. David U. Himmelstein, Terry Campbell, and Steffie Woolhandler, "Health Care Administrative Costs in the United States and Canada, 2017," *Annals of Internal Medicine*, January 7, 2020, https://doi.org/10.7326/M19-2818.
35. David U. Himmelstein et al., "A Comparison of Hospital Administrative Costs in Eight Nations: US Costs Exceed All Others by Far," *Health Affairs* 33, no. 9 (September 2014): 1586–94, https://doi.org/10.1377/hlthaff.2013.1327.
36. Julie Ann Sakowski et al., "Peering into the Black Box: Billing and Insurance Activities in a Medical Group," *Health Affairs* 28, no. 4 (July 1, 2009): w544–54, https://doi.org/10.1377/hlthaff.28.4.w544.
37. Steffie Woolhandler and David U. Himmelstein, "Single-Payer Reform: The Only Way to Fulfill the President's Pledge of More Coverage, Better Benefits, and Lower Costs," *Annals of Internal Medicine* 166, no. 8 (April 18, 2017): 587, https://doi.org/10.7326/M17-0302.
38. Uwe Reinhardt, "Where Does the Health Insurance Premium Dollar Go?," *JAMA* 317, no. 22 (June 13, 2017): 2269–70, https://doi.org/10.1001/jama.2017.6200.
39. Herbert Wiedemann, "Cleveland Clinic Letter to CMS Re: Outpatient Prospective Payment System Proposed Rule," September 26, 2019, https://www.regulations.gov/document?D=CMS-2019-0109-1814.
40. Phillip Tseng et al., "Administrative Costs Associated with Physician Billing and Insurance-Related Activities at an Academic Health Care System," *JAMA* 319, no. 7 (February 20, 2018): 691–97, https://doi.org/10.1001/jama.2017.19148.
41. Centers for Medicare and Medicaid Services, "National Health Expenditure Accounts 2018."
42. Board of Trustees, Federal Hospital Insurance and Federal Supplementary Medical Insurance Trust Funds, "2019 Annual Report of the Boards of Trustees of the Federal Hospital Insurance and Federal Supplementary Medical Insurance Trust Funds,"

April 22, 2019, https://www.cms.gov/Research-Statistics-Data-and-Systems/Statistics-Trends-and-Reports/ReportsTrustFunds/Downloads/TR2019.pdf; Kip Sullivan, "How to Think Clearly About Medicare Administrative Costs: Data Sources and Measurement," *Journal of Health Politics, Policy and Law* 38, no. 3 (June 2013): 479–504, https://doi.org/10.1215/03616878-2079523.

43. Papanicolas, Woskie, and Jha, "Health Care Spending in the United States and Other High-Income Countries."
44. Reinhardt, "Where Does the Health Insurance Premium Dollar Go?"
45. Michael Chernew et al., "Are Health Care Services Shoppable? Evidence from the Consumption of Lower-Limb MRI Scans," National Bureau of Economic Research, July 2018, https://doi.org/10.3386/w24869.
46. National Center for Health Statistics, "Health Insurance Coverage: Early Release of Estimates From the National Health Interview Survey, January-June 2019," 2019.
47. "Uninsured Rates for the Nonelderly by Race/Ethnicity," Kaiser Family Foundation, n.d., https://www.kff.org/uninsured/state-indicator/rate-by-raceethnicity.
48. "Uninsured Rates for the Nonelderly by Race/Ethnicity."
49. "Uninsured Rates for the Nonelderly by Race/Ethnicity."
50. "Uninsured Rates for the Nonelderly by Race/Ethnicity."
51. "Uninsured Rates for the Nonelderly by Race/Ethnicity."
52. Sara R. Collins, Herman K. Bhupal, and Michelle M. Doty, "Health Insurance Coverage Eight Years After the ACA: Fewer Uninsured Americans and Shorter Coverage Gaps, but More Underinsured," Commonwealth Fund, 2019, https://www.commonwealthfund.org/publications/issue-briefs/2019/feb/health-insurance-coverage-eight-years-after-aca.
53. Lydia Saad, "More Americans Delaying Medical Treatment Due to Cost," Gallup, December 9, 2019, https://news.gallup.com/poll/269138/americans-delaying-medical-treatment-due-cost.aspx.
54. G. Claxton et al., "Employer Health Benefits: 2019 Annual Survey," Kaiser Family Foundation, 2019, http://files.kff.org/attachment/Report-Employer-Health-Benefits-Annual-Survey-2019.
55. "ACA Market Unsubsidized Price Analysis," November 14, 2019, eHealthinsurance Services, Inc., https://news.ehealthinsurance.com/research/aca-market-unsubsudized-price-analysis-6782684.
56. Salam Abdus and Patricia S. Keenan, "Financial Burden of Employer-Sponsored High-Deductible Health Plans for Low-Income Adults

with Chronic Health Conditions," *JAMA Internal Medicine*, October 8, 2018, https://doi.org/10.1001/jamainternmed.2018.4706.

57. Papanicolas, Woskie, and Jha, "Health Care Spending in the United States and Other High-Income Countries."
58. Eric C. Sun et al., "Assessment of Out-of-Network Billing for Privately Insured Patients Receiving Care in In-Network Hospitals," *JAMA Internal Medicine* 179, no. 11 (2019): 1543–50, https://doi.org/10.1001/jamainternmed.2019.3451.
59. Karan R. Chhabra et al., "Out-of-Network Bills for Privately Insured Patients Undergoing Elective Surgery with In-Network Primary Surgeons and Facilities," *JAMA* 323, no. 6 (February 11, 2020): 538–47, https://doi.org/10.1001/jama.2019.21463.
60. Ashley Kirzinger, Bryan Wu, and Mollyann Brodie, "KFF Health Tracking Poll—April 2019: Surprise Medical Bills and Public's View of the Supreme Court and Continuing Protections for People with Pre-Existing Conditions," Kaiser Family Foundation, April 24, 2019, https://www.kff.org/health-costs/poll-finding/kff-health-tracking-poll-april-2019.
61. "It's Not Just the Uninsured—It's Also the Cost of Health Care," Axios, October 25, 2018, https://www.axios.com/not-just-uninsured-cost-of-health-care-cdcb4c02-0864-4e64-b745-efbe5b4b7efc.html.
62. Margot Sanger-Katz, "1,495 Americans Describe the Financial Reality of Being Really Sick," *New York Times*, October 18, 2018, https://www.nytimes.com/2018/10/17/upshot/health-insurance-severely-ill-financial-toxicity-.html.
63. "Medicare Beneficiaries' High Out-of-Pocket Costs," Commonwealth Fund, October 25, 2018, https://www.commonwealthfund.org/publications/issue-briefs/2017/may/medicare-beneficiaries-high-out-pocket-costs-cost-burdens-income.
64. Michael Anne Kyle et al., "Financial Hardships of Medicare Beneficiaries with Serious Illness," *Health Affairs* 38, no. 11 (2019): 1801–6.
65. Cassandra Yarbrough and Colin Reusch, "Progress to Build On: Recent Trends on Dental Coverage Access," *Teeth Matter: The Children's Dental Health Project's Blog*, October 18, 2018, https://www.cdhp.org/blog/557-progress-to-build-on-recent-trends-on-dental-coverage-access.
66. Karen Pollitz, Cynthia Cox, and Rachel Fehr, "Claims Denials and Appeals in ACA Marketplace Plans," Kaiser Family Foundation,

February 25, 2019, https://www.kff.org/private-insurance/issue-brief/claims-denials-and-appeals-in-aca-marketplace-plans.

67. Karen E. Joynt et al., "Hospital Closures Had No Measurable Impact on Local Hospitalization Rates or Mortality Rates, 2003–11," *Health Affairs* 34, no. 5 (May 1, 2015): 765–72, https://doi.org/10.1377/hlthaff.2014.1352.
68. "Medicaid-to-Medicare Fee Index," Kaiser Family Foundation, n.d., https://www.kff.org/medicaid/state-indicator/medicaid-to-medicare-fee-index/?currentTimeframe=0&sortModel=%7B%22colId%22:%22Location%22,%22sort%22:%22asc%22%7D; Eric Lopez, Tricia Newman, Gretchen Jacobson, et al., "How Much More Than Medicare Do Private Insurers Pay? A Review of the Literature," Kaiser Family Foundation, April 15, 2020, https://www.kff.org/medicare/issue-brief/how-much-more-than-medicare-do-private-insurers-pay-a-review-of-the-literature/.
69. Daniel Polsky et al., "Appointment Availability After Increases in Medicaid Payments for Primary Care," *New England Journal of Medicine* 372, no. 6 (February 5, 2015): 537–45, https://doi.org/10.1056/NEJMsa1413299.
70. Kaiser Family Foundation, "Primary Care Health Professional Shortage Areas (HPSAs)," September 30, 2019, https://www.kff.org/other/state-indicator/primary-care-health-professional-shortage-areas-hpsas/?currentTimeframe=0&sortModel=%7B%22colId%22:%22Location%22,%22sort%22:%22asc%22%7D#; Thomas Bodenheimer and Hoangmai H. Pham, "Primary Care: Current Problems and Proposed Solutions," *Health Affairs* 29, no. 5 (May 1, 2010): 799–805, https://doi.org/10.1377/hlthaff.2010.0026.
71. "Medscape Physician Compensation Report 2018," Medscape, October 25, 2018, https://www.medscape.com/slideshow/2018-compensation-overview-6009667.
72. Bodenheimer and Pham, "Primary Care."
73. Rachel Garfield, Gary Claxton, Anthony Damico, et al., "Eligibility for ACA Health Coverage Following Job Loss," Kaiser Family Foundation, May 13, 2020, https://www.kff.org/coronavirus-covid-19/issue-brief/eligibility-for-aca-health-coverage-following-job-loss.
74. "Job Openings and Labor Turnover—January 2020," Bureau of Labor Statistics, United States Department of Labor, March 17, 2020, https://www.bls.gov/news.release/archives/jolts_03172020.pdf.

75. Bradley Corallo and Jennifer Tolbert, "Impact of Coronavirus on Community Health Centers," Kaiser Family Foundation, May 20, 2020, https://www.kff.org/coronavirus-covid-19/issue-brief/impact-of-coronavirus-on-community-health-centers/.
76. "Employment Situation News Release," US Bureau of Labor Statistics, last modified September 23, 2020, https://www.bls.gov/news.release/archives/empsit_05082020.htm.
77. Ayla Ellison, "15 Hospitals Have Closed This Year—Here's Why," *Becker's Hospital Review*, May 15, 2020, https://www.beckershospitalreview.com/finance/15-hospitals-have-closed-this-year-here-s-why-51521.html; Ayla Ellison, "West Virginia Hospital to Close, Lay Off 340 Employees," *Becker's Hospital Review*, June 1, 2020, https://www.beckershospitalreview.com/finance/west-virginia-hospital-to-close-lay-off-340-employees.html; Sarah Kliff, "Hospitals Knew How to Make Money. Then Coronavirus Happened," *New York Times*, May 15, 2020, https://www.nytimes.com/2020/05/15/us/hospitals-revenue-coronavirus.html.
78. Sameed Ahmed M. Khatana et al., "Association of Medicaid Expansion with Cardiovascular Mortality," *JAMA Cardiology* 4, no. 7 (2019): 671–79; Sarah Miller et al., "Medicaid and Mortality: New Evidence from Linked Survey and Administrative Data," National Bureau of Economic Research, 2019, https://doi.org/10.3386/w26081.
79. Jacob Goldin, Ithai Lurie, and Janet McCubbin, "Health Insurance and Mortality: Experimental Evidence from Taxpayer Outreach," SSRN Scholarly Paper, November 26, 2019, https://papers.ssrn.com/abstract=3496282.
80. Andrew P. Wilper et al., "Health Insurance and Mortality in US Adults," *American Journal of Public Health* 99, no. 12 (December 1, 2009): 2289–95, https://doi.org/10.2105/AJPH.2008.157685; Steffie Woolhandler and David U. Himmelstein, "The Relationship of Health Insurance and Mortality: Is Lack of Insurance Deadly?," *Annals of Internal Medicine* 167, no. 6 (September 19, 2017): 424, https://doi.org/10.7326/M17-1403.
81. Jacob Bor, Gregory H. Cohen, and Sandro Galea, "Population Health in an Era of Rising Income Inequality: USA, 1980–2015," *The Lancet* 389, no. 10077 (April 2017): 1475–90, https://doi.org/10.1016/S0140-6736(17)30571-8.
82. Bor, Cohen, and Galea, "Population Health in an Era of Rising Income Inequality: USA, 1980–2015."

83. Raj Chetty et al., "The Association Between Income and Life Expectancy in the United States, 2001–2014," *JAMA* 315, no. 16 (April 26, 2016): 1750–66, https://doi.org/10.1001/jama.2016.4226.
84. Dave A. Chokshi, "Income, Poverty, and Health Inequality," *JAMA* 319, no. 13 (April 3, 2018): 1312–13, https://doi.org/10.1001/jama.2018.2521.
85. National Center for Health Statistics, "Health, United States, 2015: With Special Feature on Racial and Ethnic Health Disparities."
86. Papanicolas, Woskie, and Jha, "Health Care Spending in the United States and Other High-Income Countries."
87. E. H. Bradley et al., "Health and Social Services Expenditures: Associations with Health Outcomes," *BMJ Quality and Safety* 20, no. 10 (October 1, 2011): 826–31, https://doi.org/10.1136/bmjqs.2010.048363.
88. Irene Papanicolas et al., "The Relationship Between Health Spending and Social Spending in High-Income Countries: How Does the US Compare?," *Health Affairs* 38, no. 9 (2019): 1567–75, https://doi.org/10.1377/hlthaff.2018.05187.
89. Nia Mitchell et al., "Obesity: Overview of an Epidemic," *Psychiatric Clinics of North America* 34, no. 4 (December 2011): 717–32, https://doi.org/10.1016/j.psc.2011.08.005.
90. "Obesity Facts | Healthy Schools," CDC, January 29, 2018, https://www.cdc.gov/healthyschools/obesity/facts.htm.
91. Sarah J. Clark, Gary L. Freed, and Dianne C. Singer, "National Poll on Children's Health," C. S. Mott Children's Hospital, August 15, 2016. https://mottpoll.org/sites/default/files/documents/081516_top10.pdf.
92. Liana Fox, "The Supplemental Poverty Measure: 2018," U.S. Census Bureau, October 2019, https://www.census.gov/content/dam/Census/library/publications/2019/demo/p60-268.pdf; David U. Himmelstein et al., "Medical Bankruptcy: Still Common Despite the Affordable Care Act," *American Journal of Public Health* 109, no. 3 (February 6, 2019): 431–33, https://doi.org/10.2105/AJPH.2018.304901.
93. Larisa Antonisse et al., "The Effects of Medicaid Expansion Under the ACA: Updated Findings from a Literature Review," Kaiser Family Foundation, August 2019, https://www.kff.org/medicaid/issue-brief/the-effects-of-medicaid-expansion-under-the-aca-updated-findings-from-a-literature-review-august-2019;

Gracie Himmelstein, "Effect of the Affordable Care Act's Medicaid Expansions on Food Security, 2010–2016," *American Journal of Public Health* 109, no. 9 (2019): 1243–48, https://doi.org/10.2105/AJPH.2019.305168; Heidi L. Allen et al., "Can Medicaid Expansion Prevent Housing Evictions?," *Health Affairs* 38, no. 9 (2019): 1451–57, https://doi.org/10.1377/hlthaff.2018.05071.

94. Physicians Advocacy Institute, "Updated Physician Practice Acquisition Study: National and Regional Changes in Physician Employment, 2012–2016," March 2018, http://www.physiciansadvocacyinstitute.org/Portals/0/assets/docs/2016-PAI-Physician-Employment-Study-Final.pdf.
95. Physicians Foundation, "The Physicians Foundation 2018 Physician Survey," September 18, 2018, https://physiciansfoundation.org/wp-content/uploads/2018/09/physicians-survey-results-final-2018.pdf.
96. Physicians Foundation, "The Physicians Foundation 2018 Physician Survey."
97. Physicians Foundation, "The Physicians Foundation 2018 Physician Survey."
98. Elena Prager and Matthew Schmitt, "Employer Consolidation and Wages: Evidence from Hospitals," *SSRN Electronic Journal*, 2019, https://doi.org/10.2139/ssrn.3391889.
99. National Nurses United, "7000 Registered Nurses at 15 HCA-Affiliated Hospitals in 5 States Vote Overwhelmingly to Authorize Strike," press release, September 4, 2018, https://www.nationalnursesunited.org/press/7000-rns-15-hca-affiliated-hospitals-5-states-vote-overwhelmingly-authorize-strike.
100. Susan Houston et al., "The Intensity and Frequency of Moral Distress Among Different Healthcare Disciplines," *Journal of Clinical Ethics* 24, no. 2 (2013): 98–112.
101. Physicians Foundation, "The Physicians Foundation 2018 Physician Survey."
102. Cass Sunstein, "Wading Through the Sludge," *New York Review of Books*, April 4, 2019, https://www.nybooks.com/articles/2019/04/04/paperwork-wading-through-sludge.
103. Michael Anne Kyle and Austin Frakt, "Patient Administrative Burden in the U.S. Health Care System," unpublished manuscript, 2020.

Chapter 2

1. Irving Fisher, quoted in Jill Lepore, *These Truths: A History of the United States* (W. W. Norton, 2018), 379.
2. Paul Starr, *The Social Transformation of American Medicine: The Rise of a Sovereign Profession and the Making of a Vast Industry*, 2nd ed. (Basic Books, 2017), 245.
3. Starr, *The Social Transformation of American Medicine*, 245.
4. "Cooperation in Social Insurance Investigation," *Journal of the American Medical Association* 66, no. 19 (May 6, 1916): 1469–70, https://doi.org/10.1001/jama.1916.02580450035016.
5. "Cooperation in Social Insurance Investigation."
6. Beatrix Hoffman, *The Wages of Sickness: The Politics of Health Insurance in Progressive America* (University of North Carolina Press, 2001), 115.
7. Starr, *The Social Transformation of American Medicine*, 295.
8. Starr, *The Social Transformation of American Medicine*, 279.
9. Starr, *The Social Transformation of American Medicine*, 279.
10. Lepore, *These Truths*, 438.
11. Robert F. Wagner, "The Wagner-Murray-Dingell Bill," *Journal of the American Medical Association* 128, no. 6 (June 9, 1945): 461, https://doi.org/10.1001/jama.1945.02860230065024.
12. "Wagner-Murray-Dingell Bill for Social Security," *Journal of the American Medical Association* 122, no. 9 (June 26, 1943): 600–601, https://doi.org/10.1001/jama.1943.02840260028010; "The President's National Health Program and the New Wagner Bill," *Journal of the American Medical Association* 129, no. 14 (December 1, 1945): 950–53, https://doi.org/10.1001/jama.1945.02860480030009.
13. Starr, *The Social Transformation of American Medicine*, 283.
14. Starr, *The Social Transformation of American Medicine*, 284.
15. Lepore, *These Truths*, 547.
16. Jonathan Oberlander, *The Political Life of Medicare* (University of Chicago Press, 2003), 22.
17. Starr, *The Social Transformation of American Medicine*, 285.
18. Starr, *The Social Transformation of American Medicine*, 288.
19. Starr, *The Social Transformation of American Medicine*, 285.
20. Sven Steinmo and Jon Watts, "It's the Institutions, Stupid! Why Comprehensive National Health Insurance Always Fails in America," *Journal of Health Politics, Policy and Law* 20, no. 2 (1995): 329–72, https://doi.org/10.1215/03616878-20-2-329.

21. Robert M. Ball, "What Medicare's Architects Had in Mind," *Health Affairs* 14, no. 4 (January 1, 1995): 62–72, https://doi.org/10.1377/hlthaff.14.4.62.
22. Theodore Marmor and Jonathan Oberlander, "Medicare at Fifty," in *The Oxford Handbook of U.S. Health Law*, edited by I. Glenn Cohen, Allison K. Hoffman, and William M. Sage (Oxford University Press, 2017).
23. Theodore R. Marmor, *The Politics of Medicare* (Transaction, 1970), 13.
24. Oberlander, *The Political Life of Medicare*, 23.
25. Marmor, *The Politics of Medicare,* 32.
26. Stuart H. Altman and David Shactman, *Power, Politics, and Universal Health Care: The Inside Story of a Century-Long Battle* (Prometheus Books, 2011), 122.
27. Altman and Shactman, *Power, Politics, and Universal Health Care,* 123.
28. Richard Harris, *A Sacred Trust* (Penguin Books, 1969), 99.
29. Starr, *The Social Transformation of American Medicine*, 368.
30. Starr, *The Social Transformation of American Medicine*, 368.
31. Marmor, *The Politics of Medicare.*
32. Jill Quadagno, *One Nation, Uninsured: Why the US Has No National Health Insurance* (Oxford University Press, 2006).
33. Oberlander, *The Political Life of Medicare*, 31.
34. Paul Starr, *Remedy and Reaction: The Peculiar American Struggle over Health Care Reform* (Yale University Press, 2013).
35. Richard Nixon, Remarks at a Briefing on the Nation's Health System. Online by Gerhard Peters and John T. Woolley, The American Presidency Project https://www.presidency.ucsb.edu/node/239583.
36. Starr, *The Social Transformation of American Medicine*, 384.
37. Richard Lyons, "A Legislative Goal That Has No Foes Stalled by Differences in Approach," *New York Times*, August 27, 1974.
38. John D Wong, "IDEOLOGICAL INFLUENCE IN U.S. HEALTH POLICY: CATALYSTS OR IMPEDIMENTS?," *Journal of Health and Human Services Administration*, 1995.
39. Altman and Shactman, *Power, Politics, and Universal Health Care*, 54.
40. Uwe Reinhardt, "Medicare Innovations in the War Over the Key to the U.S. Treasury," in *Medicare and Medicaid at 50: America's Entitlement Programs in the Age of Affordable Care*, edited by Alan B. Cohen, David C. Colby, Keith A. Wailoo, and Julian E. Zelizer (Oxford University Press, 2015).

41. Starr, *The Social Transformation of American Medicine,* 463.
42. Alexis Gilman, "Preserving Competition Among Hometown Hospitals," Federal Trade Commission, March 13, 2014, https://www.ftc.gov/news-events/blogs/competition-matters/2014/03/preserving-competition-among-hometown-hospitals.
43. Rashi Fein, "What Is Wrong with the Language of Medicine?," *New England Journal of Medicine* 306, no. 14 (April 8, 1982): 863–64, https://doi.org/10.1056/NEJM198204083061409.
44. Altman and Shactman, *Power, Politics, and Universal Health Care,* 82.
45. Altman and Shactman, *Power, Politics, and Universal Health Care,* 85.
46. Altman and Shactman, *Power, Politics, and Universal Health Care,* 91.
47. Starr, *Remedy and Reaction,* 113.
48. Haynes Johnson and David S. Broder, *The System: The American Way of Politics at the Breaking Point* (Little, Brown & Co., 1996).
49. John E. McDonough, *Inside National Health Reform* (University of California Press and Milbank Memorial Fund, 2012).
50. Altman and Shactman, *Power, Politics, and Universal Health Care,* 259.
51. Altman and Shactman, *Power, Politics, and Universal Health Care,* 271.
52. Altman and Shactman, *Power, Politics, and Universal Health Care,* 264.
53. Altman and Shactman, *Power, Politics, and Universal Health Care,* 273.
54. Stuart M. Butler, "Assuring Affordable Health Care for All Americans," Heritage Foundation, 1989.
55. Ron Wyden, "Cosponsors—S.334—Healthy Americans Act," 2008, https://www.congress.gov/bill/110th-congress/senate-bill/334/cosponsors.
56. Ben Smith, "Health Reform Foes Plan Obama's 'Waterloo,'" *Politico,* July 17, 2009, https://www.politico.com/blogs/ben-smith/2009/07/health-reform-foes-plan-obamas-waterloo-019961.
57. Jennifer Tolbert et al., "Key Facts about the Uninsured Population," Kaiser Family Foundation, December 13, 2019, https://www.kff.org/uninsured/issue-brief/key-facts-about-the-uninsured-population/.
58. Edwin Bierschenk, "Woman Claims Mistreatment by Lake County Sheriff Employees," *Northwest Indiana Times,* October 10, 2014, https://www.nwitimes.com/news/local/lake/woman-claims-mistreatment-by-lake-county-sheriff-employees/article_c46c9c11-6fc8-5582-a517-5a29d6d62bdb.html.

59. Nicole Gaudiano and Maureen Groppe, "Democrats Back Medicare for All in About Half of Contested House Races," *USA Today*, October 23, 2018, https://www.usatoday.com/story/news/politics/elections/2018/10/23/democrats-back-medicare-all-half-contested-house-races/1732966002.
60. "Exit and Entrance Polls from the 2020 Primaries and Caucuses," CNN, accessed June 5, 2020, https://www.cnn.com/election/2020/entrance-and-exit-polls.
61. "Public Opinion on Single-Payer, National Health Plans, and Expanding Access to Medicare Coverage," Kaiser Family Foundation, May 27, 2020, https://www.kff.org/slideshow/public-opinion-on-single-payer-national-health-plans-and-expanding-access-to-medicare-coverage.

Chapter 3

1. "2020 Medicare Parts A & B Premiums and Deductibles," Centers for Medicare and Medicaid Services, November 8, 2019, https://www.cms.gov/newsroom/fact-sheets/2020-medicare-parts-b-premiums-and-deductibles; "High Deductible Health Plan (HDHP)," HealthCare.gov, accessed March 5, 2020, https://www.healthcare.gov/glossary/high-deductible-health-plan.
2. Cristina Boccuti et al., "Primary Care Physicians Accepting Medicare: A Snapshot," Kaiser Family Foundation, October 30, 2015, https://www.kff.org/medicare/issue-brief/primary-care-physicians-accepting-medicare-a-snapshot.
3. "Opt Out Affidavits," Centers for Medicare and Medicaid Services, January 16, 2020, https://data.cms.gov/Medicare-Enrollment/Opt-Out-Affidavits/7yuw-754z; Aaron Young et al., "FSMB Census of Licensed Physicians in the United States, 2018," *Journal of Medical Regulation* 105, no. 2 (2019): 7–23.
4. Eric Lopez, Tricia Newman, Gretchen Jacobson, et al., "How Much More Than Medicare Do Private Insurers Pay? A Review of the Literature," Kaiser Family Foundation, April 15, 2020, https://www.kff.org/medicare/issue-brief/how-much-more-than-medicare-do-private-insurers-pay-a-review-of-the-literature/.
5. Lopez, Newman, Jacobson et al., "How Much More Than Medicare Do Private Insurers Pay? A Review of the Literature."

6. Jacob Wallace and Zirui Song, "Traditional Medicare Versus Private Insurance: How Spending, Volume, And Price Change At Age Sixty-Five," *Health Affairs* 35, no. 5 (May 1, 2016): 864–72, https://doi.org/10.1377/hlthaff.2015.1195.
7. Centers for Medicare and Medicaid Services, "National Health Expenditure Accounts 2018," https://www.cms.gov/Research-Statistics-Data-and-Systems/Statistics-Trends-and-Reports/NationalHealthExpendData/NationalHealthAccountsHistorical, accessed March 4, 2020; Board of Trustees, Federal Hospital Insurance and Federal Supplementary Medical Insurance Trust Funds, "2019 Annual Report of the Boards of Trustees of the Federal Hospital Insurance and Federal Supplementary Medical Insurance Trust Funds," April 22, 2019, https://www.cms.gov/Research-Statistics-Data-and-Systems/Statistics-Trends-and-Reports/ReportsTrustFunds/Downloads/TR2019.pdf.
8. Gary Claxton, Bradley Sawyer, and Cynthia Cox, "How Affordability of Health Care Varies by Income Among People with Employer Coverage," Peterson-Kaiser Health System Tracker, April 14, 2019, https://www.healthsystemtracker.org/brief/how-affordability-of-health-care-varies-by-income-among-people-with-employer-coverage.
9. Note that in this book we use "public good" in its ordinary sense (i.e., a good or service made available without profit to all members of the public), rather than the economists' technical sense of a nonrival and nonexcludable good.
10. Thomas M. Selden et al., "The Growing Difference Between Public and Private Payment Rates for Inpatient Hospital Care," *Health Affairs* 34, no. 12 (December 2015): 2147–50, https://doi.org/10.1377/hlthaff.2015.0706.
11. Drew Altman, "Private Insurance's Costs Are Skyrocketing," Axios, December 16, 2019, https://www.axios.com/health-insurance-costs-private-medicare-medicaid-c40bb6f1-c638-4bc3-9a71-c1787829e62e.html.
12. David U. Himmelstein, Terry Campbell, and Steffie Woolhandler, "Health Care Administrative Costs in the United States and Canada, 2017," *Annals of Internal Medicine*, January 7, 2020, https://doi.org/10.7326/M19-2818.
13. Centers for Medicare and Medicaid Services, "National Health Expenditure Accounts 2018."
14. Board of Trustees, Federal Hospital Insurance and Federal Supplementary Medical Insurance Trust Funds, "2019 Annual

Report of the Boards of Trustees of the Federal Hospital Insurance and Federal Supplementary Medical Insurance Trust Funds," April 22, 2019, https://www.cms.gov/Research-Statistics-Data-and-Systems/Statistics-Trends-and-Reports/ReportsTrustFunds/Downloads/TR2019.pdf.

15. Critics sometimes claim that Medicare's administrative costs appear low as a percentage of program spending merely because Medicare beneficiaries have higher total spending than their younger peers. This claim is contradicted by evidence that Medicare Advantage plans have administrative costs nearly identical to other private insurance plans, despite covering a similar population as the traditional Medicare program. For further discussion of administrative costs in Medicare for All, see Appendix A in Donald Berwick and Simon Johnson, "Warren Medicare for All Plan Cost Estimate Letter," October 31, 2019, https://assets.ctfassets.net/4ubxbgy9463z/2Tg9oB55ICu2vtYBaKKcVr/d124e0eeb128ad3a8d8ab8a6ccae44c0/20191031_Medicare_for_All_Cost_Letter___Appendices_FINAL.pdf.
16. Himmelstein, Campbell, and Woolhandler, "Health Care Administrative Costs in the United States and Canada, 2017."
17. Brett Venker, Kevin B. Stephenson, and Walid F. Gellad, "Assessment of Spending in Medicare Part D if Medication Prices from the Department of Veterans Affairs Were Used," *JAMA Internal Medicine* 179, no. 3 (March 1, 2019): 431–33, https://doi.org/10.1001/jamainternmed.2018.5874.
18. Lunna Lopes et al., "Data Note: Public Worries About and Experience with Surprise Medical Bills," Kaiser Family Foundation, February 28, 2020, https://www.kff.org/health-costs/poll-finding/data-note-public-worries-about-and-experience-with-surprise-medical-bills.
19. Alison P. Galvani et al., "Improving the Prognosis of Health Care in the USA," *The Lancet* 395, no. 10223 (February 15, 2020): 524–33, https://doi.org/10.1016/S0140-6736(19)33019-3.
20. Liana Fox, "The Supplemental Poverty Measure: 2018," U.S. Census Bureau, October 2019, https://www.census.gov/content/dam/Census/library/publications/2019/demo/p60-268.pdf.
21. "Blood Pressure Medicines for Five Years to Prevent Death, Heart Attacks, and Strokes," The NNT Group, July 21, 2014, https://www.thennt.com/nnt/anti-hypertensives-to-prevent-death-heart-attacks-and-strokes/.
22. Brendan Murphy, "For First Time, Physician Practice Owners Are Not the Majority," American Medical Association, May 31, 2017,

https://www.ama-assn.org/practice-management/economics/first-time-physician-practice-owners-are-not-majority.

23. Christine Sinsky et al., "Allocation of Physician Time in Ambulatory Practice: A Time and Motion Study in 4 Specialties," *Annals of Internal Medicine* 165, no. 11 (2016): 753–60.
24. N. Lance Downing, David W. Bates, and Christopher A. Longhurst, "Physician Burnout in the Electronic Health Record Era: Are We Ignoring the Real Cause?," *Annals of Internal Medicine* 169, no. 1 (July 3, 2018): 50, https://doi.org/10.7326/M18-0139.

Chapter 4

1. David Grabowski, Jonathan Gruber, and Vincent Mor, "You're Probably Going to Need Medicaid," *New York Times*, January 20, 2018, https://www.nytimes.com/2017/06/13/opinion/youre-probably-going-to-need-medicaid.html.
2. Grabowski, Gruber, and Mor, "You're Probably Going to Need Medicaid."
3. Jill Quadagno, *One Nation, Uninsured: Why the US Has No National Health Insurance* (Oxford University Press, 2006).
4. Elizabeth Warren, "Ending the Stranglehold of Health Care Costs on American Families," n.d., https://elizabethwarren.com/plans/paying-for-m4a.
5. Leah Zallman et al., "Immigrants Contributed an Estimated $115.2 Billion More to the Medicare Trust Fund than They Took out in 2002–09," *Health Affairs* 32, no. 6 (2013): 1153–60.
6. Leah Zallman et al., "Immigrants Pay More in Private Insurance Premiums Than They Receive in Benefits," *Health Affairs* 37, no. 10 (October 2018): 1663–68, https://doi.org/10.1377/hlthaff.2018.0309.
7. Katherine Baicker and Dana Goldman, "Patient Cost-Sharing and Healthcare Spending Growth," *Journal of Economic Perspectives* 25, no. 2 (May 2011): 47–68, https://doi.org/10.1257/jep.25.2.47.
8. Zarek C. Brot-Goldberg et al., "What Does a Deductible Do? The Impact of Cost-Sharing on Health Care Prices, Quantities, and Spending Dynamics," *Quarterly Journal of Economics* 132, no. 3 (August 1, 2017): 1261–318, https://doi.org/10.1093/qje/qjx013.
9. J. Frank Wharam et al., "Vulnerable and Less Vulnerable Women in High-Deductible Health Plans Experienced Delayed Breast Cancer

Care," *Health Affairs* 38, no. 3 (March 1, 2019): 408–15, https://doi.org/10.1377/hlthaff.2018.05026.

10. Robert H. Brook et al., "The Health Insurance Experiment: A Classic RAND Study Speaks to the Current Health Care Reform Debate," RAND Corporation, 2006, https://www.rand.org/pubs/research_briefs/RB9174.html.
11. Ashley Kirzinger et al., "KFF Health Tracking Poll—February 2019: Prescription Drugs," Kaiser Family Foundation, March 1, 2019, https://www.kff.org/health-costs/poll-finding/kff-health-tracking-poll-february-2019-prescription-drugs.
12. Niteesh K. Choudhry et al., "Full Coverage for Preventive Medications After Myocardial Infarction," *New England Journal of Medicine* 365, no. 22 (December 1, 2011): 2088–97, https://doi.org/10.1056/NEJMsa1107913.
13. Julia Thornton Snider et al., "Impact of Type 2 Diabetes Medication Cost Sharing on Patient Outcomes and Health Plan Costs," *American Journal of Managed Care* 22, no. 6 (2016): 433–40.
14. Austin Frakt and Aaron E. Carroll, "Build Your Own 'Medicare for All' Plan. Beware: There Are Tough Choices," *New York Times*, February 21, 2019, https://www.nytimes.com/interactive/2019/02/21/upshot/up-medicareforall.html.
15. Jeffrey Peppercorn et al., "Impact of the Elimination of Cost Sharing for Mammographic Breast Cancer Screening Among Rural US Women: A Natural Experiment," *Cancer* 123, no. 13 (July 1, 2017): 2506–15, https://doi.org/10.1002/cncr.30629; Xuesong Han et al., "Has Recommended Preventive Service Use Increased After Elimination of Cost-Sharing as Part of the Affordable Care Act in the United States?," *Preventive Medicine* 78 (September 2015): 85–91, https://doi.org/10.1016/j.ypmed.2015.07.012.
16. Rajender Agarwal, Olena Mazurenko, and Nir Menachemi, "High-Deductible Health Plans Reduce Health Care Cost and Utilization, Including Use of Needed Preventive Services," *Health Affairs* 36, no. 10 (October 2017): 1762–68, https://doi.org/10.1377/hlthaff.2017.0610.
17. Marika Cabral and Mark R. Cullen, "The Effect of Insurance Coverage on Preventive Care," *Economic Inquiry* 55, no. 3 (July 2017): 1452–67, https://doi.org/10.1111/ecin.12442.

18. Kaiser Family Foundation, "An Overview of Medicare," February 2019, https://www.kff.org/medicare/issue-brief/an-overview-of-medicare.
19. "2018 Medicare Supplement Loss Ratios," National Association of Insurance Commissioners, 2019, https://naic.org/prod_serv/MED-BB-19.pdf.
20. Jenny Gold, "Obamacare's Cost-Control Programs May Be Contagious," *Washington Post*, August 29, 2013, https://www.washingtonpost.com/news/wonk/wp/2013/08/29/obamacares-cost-control-programs-may-be-contagious.
21. Michael L. Barnett et al., "Two-Year Evaluation of Mandatory Bundled Payments for Joint Replacement," *New England Journal of Medicine* 380, no. 3 (2019): 252–62, https://doi.org/10.1056/NEJMsa1809010; J. Michael McWilliams et al., "Medicare Spending After 3 Years of the Medicare Shared Savings Program," *New England Journal of Medicine* 379, no. 12 (September 20, 2018): 1139–49, https://doi.org/10.1056/NEJMsa1803388; Austin B. Frakt and Ashish K. Jha, "Face the Facts: We Need to Change the Way We Do Pay for Performance," *Annals of Internal Medicine* 168, no. 4 (February 20, 2018): 291, https://doi.org/10.7326/M17-3005.
22. Jonathan E. Fried, David T. Liebers, and Eric T. Roberts, "Sustaining Rural Hospitals After COVID-19: The Case for Global Budgets," *JAMA* 324, no. 2 (July 14, 2020): 137–38, https://doi.org/10.1001/jama.2020.9744.
23. Zirui Song et al., "Health Care Spending, Utilization, and Quality 8 Years into Global Payment," *New England Journal of Medicine* 381, no. 3 (July 18, 2019): 252–63, https://doi.org/10.1056/NEJMsa1813621.
24. Micah Johnson, Sanjay Kishore, and Donald M. Berwick, "Medicare for All: An Analysis of Key Policy Issues.," *Health Affairs (Project Hope)* 39, no. 1 (2020): 133–41.
25. Johnson, Kishore, and Berwick, "Medicare for All."
26. "Health Care Spending and the Medicare Program," MedPAC, 2019, http://www.medpac.gov/docs/default-source/data-book/jun19_databook_entirereport_sec.pdf?sfvrsn=0.
27. "Medicaid-to-Medicare Fee Index," Kaiser Family Foundation, n.d., https://www.kff.org/medicaid/state-indicator/medicaid-to-medicare-fee-index/.

28. Robert Pollin et al., "Economic Analysis of Medicare for All," Political Economy Research Institute, University of Massachusetts, Amherst, 2018, https://www.peri.umass.edu/publication/item/download/805_42f6acc20a83c79049e68b270e30ee43.
29. "Poll: Nearly 1 in 4 Americans Taking Prescription Drugs Say It's Difficult to Afford Their Medicines, Including Larger Shares Among Those with Health Issues, with Low Incomes and Nearing Medicare Age," Kaiser Family Foundation, March 1, 2019, https://www.kff.org/health-costs/press-release/poll-nearly-1-in-4-americans-taking-prescription-drugs-say-its-difficult-to-afford-medicines-including-larger-shares-with-low-incomes.
30. "Striking a 'Grand Bargain' for a PCSK9 Inhibitor," Institute for Clinical and Economic Review, May 2, 2018, https://icer-review.org/blog/pcsk9-grand-bargain.
31. "Striking a 'Grand Bargain' for a PCSK9 Inhibitor."
32. Sy Mukherjee, "Protect at All Costs: How the Maker of the World's Bestselling Drug Keeps Prices Sky-High," *Fortune*, July 18, 2019, https://fortune.com/longform/abbvie-humira-drug-costs-innovation.
33. Mukherjee, "Protect at All Costs: How the Maker of the World's Bestselling Drug Keeps Prices Sky-High."
34. Andrew Dunn, "With Boehringer Settlement, AbbVie Completes Humira Sweep," Biopharma Dive, May 14, 2019, https://www.biopharmadive.com/news/abbvie-boehringer-ingelheim-settle-humira-patent-biosimilar/554729.
35. James Love, "Evidence Regarding Research and Development Investments in Innovative and Non-Innovative Medicines," Consumer Project on Technology, 2003, 22, http://www.cptech.org/ip/health/rnd/evidenceregardingrnd.pdf.
36. Aaron S. Kesselheim, Jerry Avorn, and Ameet Sarpatwari, "The High Cost of Prescription Drugs in the United States: Origins and Prospects for Reform," *JAMA* 316, no. 8 (August 23, 2016): 858, https://doi.org/10.1001/jama.2016.11237.
37. Rahul K. Nayak, Jerry Avorn, and Aaron S. Kesselheim, "Public Sector Financial Support for Late Stage Discovery of New Drugs in the United States: Cohort Study," *BMJ (Clinical Research Ed.)* 367, no. 23 (2019): 15766, https://doi.org/10.1136/bmj.l5766.
38. Andrew C. Singer, Claas Kirchhelle, and Adam P. Roberts, "Reinventing the Antimicrobial Pipeline in Response to the Global

Crisis of Antimicrobial-Resistant Infections," *F1000Research* 8 (March 1, 2019), https://doi.org/10.12688/f1000research.18302.1.

39. Medicaid and CHIP Payment and Access Commission, *Medicaid's Role in Disasters and Public Health Emergencies* (Washington, DC: MACPAC, 2018), https://www.macpac.gov/wp-content/uploads/2018/03/Medicaid%E2%80%99s-Role-in-Disasters-and-Public-Health-Emergencies.pdf.

Chapter 5

1. Katherine Grace Carman, Jodi Liu, and Chapin White, "Accounting for the Burden and Redistribution of Health Care Costs: Who Uses Care and Who Pays for It," *Health Services Research*, January 28, 2020, https://doi.org/10.1111/1475-6773.13258.
2. Carman, Liu, and White, "Accounting for the Burden and Redistribution of Health Care Costs."
3. Carman, Liu, and White, "Accounting for the Burden and Redistribution of Health Care Costs."
4. Paul D. Jacobs and Thomas M. Selden, "Changes in the Equity of US Health Care Financing in the Period 2005–16," *Health Affairs* 38, no. 11 (October 16, 2019): 1791–800, https://doi.org/10.1377/hlthaff.2019.00625.
5. Carman, Liu, and White, "Accounting for the Burden and Redistribution of Health Care Costs."
6. Jacobs and Selden, "Changes in the Equity of US Health Care Financing in the Period 2005–16."
7. "Out-of-Pocket Spending," Peterson-Kaiser Health System Tracker, December 24, 2019, https://www.healthsystemtracker.org/indicator/access-affordability/out-of-pocket-spending.
8. Charles Blahous, "The Costs of a National Single-Payer Healthcare System," Mercatus Center at George Mason University, July 2018, https://www.mercatus.org/system/files/blahous-costs-medicare-mercatus-working-paper-v1_1.pdf.
9. Linda J. Blumberg, John Holahan, and Michael Simpson, "Don't Confuse Changes in Federal Health Spending with National Health Spending," Urban Institute, October 16, 2019, https://www.urban.org/urban-wire/dont-confuse-changes-federal-health-spending-national-health-spending.
10. Donald Berwick and Simon Johnson, "Warren Medicare for All Plan Cost Estimate Letter," October 31, 2019, https://assets.

ctfassets.net/4ubxbgy9463z/2Tg9oB55ICu2vtYBaKKcVr/d124e0eeb128ad3a8d8ab8a6ccae44c0/20191031_Medicare_for_All_Cost_Letter___Appendices_FINAL.pdf; Alison P. Galvani et al., "Improving the Prognosis of Health Care in the USA," *The Lancet* 395, no. 10223 (February 15, 2020): 524–33, https://doi.org/10.1016/S0140-6736(19)33019-3; "Primary Care: Estimating Leading Democratic Candidates' Health Plans," Committee for a Responsible Federal Budget, January 24, 2020, http://www.crfb.org/sites/default/files/Primary_Care_Estimating_Leading_Democratic_Candidates_Health_Plans.pdf; John Holahan et al., "The Sanders Single-Payer Health Care Plan," Urban Institute, 2016, https://www.urban.org/research/publication/sanders-single-payer-health-care-plan-effect-national-health-expenditures-and-federal-and-private-spending; Linda J. Blumberg et al., "From Incremental to Comprehensive Health Insurance Reform: How Various Reform Options Compare on Coverage and Costs," Urban Institute, October 16, 2019, 81; Blahous, "The Costs of a National Single-Payer Healthcare System"; Jodi Liu and Christine Eibner, "National Health Spending Estimates Under Medicare for All," RAND Corporation, 2019, https://www.rand.org/pubs/research_reports/RR3106.html; Gerald Friedman, "Yes, We Can Have Improved Medicare for All," Hopbrook Institute, March 2019, https://f411bec1-69cf-4acb-bb86-370f4ddb5cba.filesusr.com/ugd/698411_9144a6d2d0374ec1a183b30e8369738b.pdf; Kenneth E. Thorpe, "An Analysis of Senator Sanders['s] Single Payer Plan," Emory University, January 27, 2016, https://www.healthcare-now.org/296831690-Kenneth-Thorpe-s-analysis-of-Bernie-Sanders-s-single-payer-proposal.pdf; Robert Pollin et al., "Economic Analysis of Medicare for All," Political Economy Research Institute, University of Massachusetts, Amherst, 2018, https://www.peri.umass.edu/publication/item/download/805_42f6acc20a83c79049e68b270e30ee43.

11. Christopher Cai et al., "Projected Costs of Single-Payer Healthcare Financing in the United States: A Systematic Review of Economic Analyses," *PLOS Medicine* 17, no. 1 (January 15, 2020): e1003013, https://doi.org/10.1371/journal.pmed.1003013.
12. Rabah Kamal, Daniel McDermott, and Cynthia Cox, "How Has U.S. Spending on Healthcare Changed over Time?," Peterson-Kaiser Health System Tracker, December 20, 2019, https://www.

healthsystemtracker.org/chart-collection/u-s-spending-healthcare-changed-time.

13. Thomas M. Selden et al., "The Growing Difference Between Public and Private Payment Rates for Inpatient Hospital Care," *Health Affairs* 34, no. 12 (December 2015): 2147–50, https://doi.org/10.1377/hlthaff.2015.0706.
14. The Committee for a Responsible Federal Budget (CRFB) later conducted their own assessment of Warren's plan. The spending estimates given by the Warren campaign fell between the low and central estimates given by CRFB for the projected costs of the plan, reflecting uncertainty on issues including utilization increases, drug price reductions, and the rate of spending growth over time. "Primary Care: Estimating Leading Democratic Candidates' Health Plans"; "Warren Medicare for All Plan Cost Estimate Letter."
15. Thomas Kaplan, Abby Goodnough, and Margot Sanger-Katz, "Elizabeth Warren Proposes $20.5 Trillion Health Care Plan," *New York Times*, November 1, 2019, https://www.nytimes.com/2019/11/01/us/politics/elizabeth-warren-medicare-for-all.html.
16. David U. Himmelstein, Terry Campbell, and Steffie Woolhandler, "Health Care Administrative Costs in the United States and Canada, 2017," *Annals of Internal Medicine*, January 7, 2020, https://doi.org/10.7326/M19-2818.
17. Micah Johnson, Sanjay Kishore, and Donald M. Berwick, "Medicare for All: An Analysis of Key Policy Issues.," *Health Affairs (Project Hope)* 39, no. 1 (2020): 133–41.
18. "Federal Subsidies for Health Insurance Coverage for People Under Age 65: 2017 to 2027," Congressional Budget Office, September 2017.
19. Andrew Sprung, "98% of Americans with Health Insurance Are Subsidized. How Bout the Other 2%?," *Xpostfactoid: Mostly About the ACA: Obamacare to Trumpcare* (blog), May 25, 2016, https://xpostfactoid.blogspot.com/2016/05/98-of-americans-with-health-insurance.html.
20. Gary Claxton, Bradley Sawyer, and Cynthia Cox, "How Affordability of Health Care Varies by Income Among People with Employer Coverage," Peterson-Kaiser Health System Tracker, April 14, 2019, https://www.healthsystemtracker.org/brief/how-affordability-of-health-care-varies-by-income-among-people-with-employer-coverage.

21. "How Does Bernie Pay for His Major Plans?," Bernie Sanders Official Campaign Website, 2020, https://berniesanders.com/issues/how-does-bernie-pay-his-major-plans.
22. Elizabeth Warren, "Ending the Stranglehold of Health Care Costs on American Families," n.d., https://elizabethwarren.com/plans/paying-for-m4a.
23. Jodi Liu et al., *An Assessment of the New York Health Act: A Single-Payer Option for New York State* (RAND Corporation, 2018), https://www.rand.org/content/dam/rand/pubs/research_reports/RR2400/RR2424/RAND_RR2424.pdf.
24. Larry DeWitt, "Research Note #23: Luther Gulick Memorandum Re: Famous FDR Quote," Research Notes and Special Studies by the SSA Historian's Office, July 21, 2005, https://www.ssa.gov/history/Gulick.html.

Chapter 6

1. Jennifer Tolbert et al., "Key Facts About the Uninsured Population," Kaiser Family Foundation, December 13, 2019, https://www.kff.org/uninsured/issue-brief/key-facts-about-the-uninsured-population.
2. Matthew Fiedler et al., "Building on the ACA to Achieve Universal Coverage," *New England Journal of Medicine* 380, no. 18 (May 2, 2019): 1685–88, https://doi.org/10.1056/NEJMp1901532.
3. "Health Insurance Coverage of the Total Population," Kaiser Family Foundation, 2019, https://www.kff.org/other/state-indicator/total-population/?currentTimeframe=0&sortModel=%7B%22colId%22:%22Uninsured%22,%22sort%22:%22asc%22%7D.
4. Brent D. Fulton, "Health Care Market Concentration Trends in the United States: Evidence and Policy Responses," *Health Affairs* 36, no. 9 (September 2017): 1530–38, https://doi.org/10.1377/hlthaff.2017.0556.
5. "Health Insurance Coverage of Nonelderly 0–64," Kaiser Family Foundation, 2018, https://www.kff.org/other/state-indicator/nonelderly-0-64/?currentTimeframe=0&sortModel=%7B%22colId%22%3A%22Uninsured%22%2C%22sort%22%3A%22asc%22%7D.
6. AFL-CIO and National Nurses United, "Taking Neighbors to Court: Johns Hopkins Hospital Medical Debt Lawsuits," May 2019, https://act.nationalnursesunited.org/page/-/files/graphics/Johns-Hopkins-Medical-Debt-report.pdf.

7. Urban Institute, "Debt in America: An Interactive Map," December 17, 2019, https://apps.urban.org/features/debt-interactive-map/?type=overall&variable=pct_w_medical_debt_in_collections.
8. "Add a 'Public Plan' to the Health Insurance Exchanges," Congressional Budget Office, November 2013, https://www.cbo.gov/budget-options/2013/44890.
9. Rosa L. DeLauro, "Medicare for America Act of 2019," Pub. L. No. H.R.2452 (2019), https://www.congress.gov/bill/116th-congress/house-bill/2452.
10. DeLauro, "Medicare for America Act of 2019."
11. Medicare Payment Advisory Commission, "Report to the Congress: Medicare Payment Policy," March 2019.
12. Juliette Cubanski, Tricia Neuman, and Meredith Freed, "The Facts on Medicare Spending and Financing," Kaiser Family Foundation, August 20, 2019, https://www.kff.org/medicare/issue-brief/the-facts-on-medicare-spending-and-financing.
13. David J. Meyers et al., "Analysis of Drivers of Disenrollment and Plan Switching Among Medicare Advantage Beneficiaries," *JAMA Internal Medicine* 179, no. 4 (April 1, 2019): 524–32, https://doi.org/10.1001/jamainternmed.2018.7639.
14. Gretchen Jacobson, Tricia Neuman, and Anthony Damico, "Do People Who Sign Up for Medicare Advantage Plans Have Lower Medicare Spending?," Kaiser Family Foundation, May 7, 2019, https://www.kff.org/report-section/do-people-who-sign-up-for-medicare-advantage-plans-have-lower-medicare-spending-issue-brief.
15. Hailey Mensik, "DOJ sues Cigna, alleging $1.4B in Medicare Advantage fraud," August 6, 2020, https://www.healthcaredive.com/news/doj-cigna-medicare-advantage-fraud-lawsuit/583023/; Kelsey Waddill, "DOJ Launches Lawsuit Against Anthem for Risk Adjustment Fraud," March 30, 2020, https://healthpayerintelligence.com/news/doj-launches-lawsuit-against-anthem-for-risk-adjustment-fraud
16. Steffie Woolhandler and David U. Himmelstein, "The American College of Physicians' Endorsement of Single-Payer Reform: A Sea Change for the Medical Profession," *Annals of Internal Medicine* 172, no. 2 supp. (January 21, 2020): S60, https://doi.org/10.7326/M19-3775.
17. Bradley Sawyer and Gary Claxton, "How Do Health Expenditures Vary Across the Population?," Peterson-Kaiser Health System Tracker, January 16, 2019, https://www.healthsystemtracker.org/chart-collection/health-expenditures-vary-across-population.

Chapter 7

1. Amina Dunn, "Democrats Differ over Best Way to Provide Health Coverage for All Americans," Pew Research Center, July 26, 2019, https://www.pewresearch.org/fact-tank/2019/07/26/democrats-differ-over-best-way-to-provide-health-coverage-for-all-americans.
2. Ashley Kirzinger, Bryan Wu, and Mollyann Brodie, "Kaiser Health Tracking Poll—March 2018: Views on Prescription Drug Pricing and Medicare-for-All Proposals," March 23, 2018, https://www.kff.org/health-costs/poll-finding/kaiser-health-tracking-poll-march-2018-prescription-drug-pricing-medicare-for-all-proposals.
3. Yusra Murad, "Majority of Voters Back National Health Plan—Unless It's Called 'Single Payer,'" Morning Consult, November 29, 2018, https://morningconsult.com/2018/11/29/majority-of-voters-back-national-health-plan-unless-its-called-single-payer.
4. "Exit and Entrance Polls from the 2020 Primaries and Caucuses," CNN, accessed June 5, 2020, https://www.cnn.com/election/2020/entrance-and-exit-polls.
5. Jake Johnson, "As Centrist Democrat Who Lost Reelection Attacks Medicare for All, Progressives Respond with the Facts," Common Dreams, December 30, 2018, https://www.commondreams.org/news/2018/12/30/centrist-democrat-who-lost-reelection-attacks-medicare-all-progressives-respond.
6. "Future of the Party Report," Data for Progress, accessed March 9, 2020, https://www.dataforprogress.org/future-of-the-party-report.
7. Laura Wronski, "New York Times SurveyMonkey Poll: November 2019," SurveyMonkey, accessed February 28, 2020, https://www.surveymonkey.com/curiosity/nyt-november-2019-cci.
8. Wronski, "New York Times SurveyMonkey Poll."
9. Ashley Kirzinger et al., "Kaiser Health Tracking Poll—June 2017: ACA, Replacement Plan, and Medicaid," Kaiser Family Foundation, June 23, 2017, https://www.kff.org/health-reform/poll-finding/kaiser-health-tracking-poll-june-2017-aca-replacement-plan-and-medicaid.
10. "Public Opinion on Single-Payer, National Health Plans, and Expanding Access to Medicare Coverage," Kaiser Family Foundation, May 27, 2020, https://www.kff.org/slideshow/public-opinion-on-single-payer-national-health-plans-and-expanding-access-to-medicare-coverage.

11. John Cawley, Asako S. Moriya, and Kosali I. Simon, "The Impact of the Macroeconomy on Health Insurance Coverage: Evidence from the Great Recession," Working Paper, National Bureau of Economic Research, November 2011, https://doi.org/10.3386/w17600.
12. John Holahan, "The 2007–09 Recession and Health Insurance Coverage," *Health Affairs* 30, no. 1 (January 1, 2011): 145–52, https://doi.org/10.1377/hlthaff.2010.1003.
13. "U.S. House Election Results 2018," *New York Times*, November 6, 2018, https://www.nytimes.com/interactive/2018/11/06/us/elections/results-house-elections.html.
14. "CNN 2018 Midterms Exit Polling," 2018, https://www.cnn.com/election/2018/exit-polls.
15. "Benchmark Employer Survey Finds Average Family Premiums Now Top $20,000," Kaiser Family Foundation, September 25, 2019, https://www.kff.org/health-costs/press-release/benchmark-employer-survey-finds-average-family-premiums-now-top-20000.
16. Gary Claxton et al., "Employer Health Benefits: 2009 Annual Survey," Kaiser Family Foundation and Health Research and Educational Trust, 2009, https://www.kff.org/wp-content/uploads/2013/04/7936.pdf; G. Claxton et al., "Employer Health Benefits: 2019 Annual Survey," Kaiser Family Foundation, 2019, http://files.kff.org/attachment/Report-Employer-Health-Benefits-Annual-Survey-2019.
17. Eric C. Sun et al., "Assessment of Out-of-Network Billing for Privately Insured Patients Receiving Care in In-Network Hospitals," *JAMA Internal Medicine* 179, no. 11 (2019): 1543–50, https://doi.org/10.1001/jamainternmed.2019.3451.
18. Stan Dorn, "The COVID-19 Pandemic and Resulting Economic Crash Have Caused the Greatest Health Insurance Losses in American History," Families USA, July 13, 2020, https://www.familiesusa.org/resources/the-covid-19-pandemic-and-resulting-economic-crash-have-caused-the-greatest-health-insurance-losses-in-american-history.
19. Adrianna McIntyre et al., "The Affordable Care Act's Missing Consensus: Values, Attitudes, and Experiences Associated with Competing Health Reform Preferences," *Journal of Health Politics, Policy and Law*, 45, no. 5 (October 1, 2020): 729–55, https://doi.org/10.1215/03616878-8543222.
20. Yusra Murad, "As Coronavirus Surges, 'Medicare for All' Support Hits 9-Month High," Morning Consult, April 1, 2020,

https://morningconsult.com/2020/04/01/medicare-for-all-coronavirus-pandemic.

21. Rashi Fein, *Medical Care, Medical Costs: The Search for a Health Insurance Policy* (Harvard University Press, 1986), 151.
22. Kaiser Family Foundation, "Public Opinion on Single-Payer, National Health Plans, and Expanding Access to Medicare Coverage."
23. Kaiser Family Foundation, "Public Opinion on Single-Payer, National Health Plans, and Expanding Access to Medicare Coverage."
24. Ricardo Alonso-Zaldivar, "People Love Medicare for All Until They're Told It'll Raise Taxes," *Business Insider*, January 26, 2019, https://www.businessinsider.com/ap-poll-support-for-medicare-for-all-fluctuates-with-details-2019-1.
25. Ashley Kirzinger, Cailey Muñana, and Mollyann Brodie, "KFF Health Tracking Poll—January 2019: The Public on Next Steps for the ACA and Proposals to Expand Coverage," Kaiser Family Foundation, January 23, 2019, https://www.kff.org/health-reform/poll-finding/kff-health-tracking-poll-january-2019.
26. Lunna Lopes et al., "KFF Health Tracking Poll—November 2019: Health Care in the 2020 Election, Medicare-for-All, and the State of the ACA," Kaiser Family Foundation, November 20, 2019, https://www.kff.org/health-reform/poll-finding/kff-health-tracking-poll-november-2019.
27. Sean McElwee and John Ray, "Polling on Medicare for All," Data for Progress, 2019, http://filesforprogress.org/memos/medicare-for-all-polling.pdf.
28. Ian Snively, "Rep. Andy Harris: 'If You Like the DMV, You'll Love Medicare for All,'" Townhall, March 6, 2019, https://townhall.com/tipsheet/iansnively/2019/03/06/if-you-like-the-dmv-youll-love-medicare-for-all-conservative-congressman-says-n2542707.
29. Insurance Information Institute, "Facts + Statistics: Insurance Industry Overview," 2019, https://www.iii.org/fact-statistic/facts-statistics-industry-overview; Robert Pollin et al., "Economic Analysis of Medicare for All," Political Economy Research Institute, University of Massachusetts, Amherst, 2018, https://www.peri.umass.edu/publication/item/download/805_42f6acc20a83c79049e68b270e30ee43.

Chapter 8

1. R. J. Reinhart, "Nurses Continue to Rate Highest in Honesty, Ethics," Gallup, January 6, 2020, https://news.gallup.com/poll/274673/nurses-continue-rate-highest-honesty-ethics.aspx.
2. "Top Lobbying Industries in the United States in 2018, by Total Lobbying Spending," Statista, March 2019, https://www.statista.com/statistics/257364/top-lobbying-industries-in-the-us.
3. "Industries," Center for Responsive Politics, 2019, https://www.opensecrets.org/federal-lobbying/industries?cycle=a.
4. "Top Spenders: 2019," Center for Responsive Politics, 2020, https://www.opensecrets.org/federal-lobbying/top-spenders?cycle=2019.
5. Lindsay Resnick, "Get Ready for a Future of Rampant Healthcare Consolidation," *Becker's Hospital Review*, August 7, 2018, https://www.beckershospitalreview.com/healthcare-information-technology/get-ready-for-a-future-of-rampant-healthcare-consolidation.html.
6. "The Great Consolidation: The Potential for Rapid Consolidation of Health Systems," Deloitte United States, accessed February 16, 2020, https://www2.deloitte.com/us/en/pages/life-sciences-and-health-care/articles/great-consolidation-health-systems.html.
7. Joe Cantlupe, "Number of Healthcare Administrators Explodes Since 1970," Athena Health, November 7, 2017, https://www.athenahealth.com/knowledge-hub/practice-management/expert-forum-rise-and-rise-healthcare-administrator.
8. Centers for Medicare and Medicaid Services, "National Health Expenditure Accounts 2018," https://www.cms.gov/Research-Statistics-Data-and-Systems/Statistics-Trends-and-Reports/NationalHealthExpendData/NationalHealthAccountsHistorical, accessed March 4, 2020.
9. Cyrus Moulton, "UMass CEO Eric Dickson Backs Medicare for All, Calls Plan 'Bold, Courageous,'" *Telegram and Gazette* (Worcester, MA), December 7, 2019, https://www.telegram.com/news/20191207/umass-ceo-eric-dickson-backs-medicare-for-all-calls-plan-bold-courageous.
10. Adam Cancryn and Rachel Roubein, "'Medicare for All' Backers Find Biggest Foe in Their Own Backyard," Politico, May 25, 2019, https://politi.co/2wlwOKx.
11. Justin McCarthy, "Big Pharma Sinks to the Bottom of U.S. Industry Rankings," Gallup, September 3, 2019, https://news.

gallup.com/poll/266060/big-pharma-sinks-bottom-industry-rankings.aspx.

12. Cancryn and Roubein, "'Medicare for All' Backers Find Biggest Foe in Their Own Backyard."
13. Letter from Melanie Sloan, exective director of Citizens for Responsibility and Ethics in Washington, to Mark T. Bertolini, chairman and CEO of Aetna, June 14, 2012, https://s3.amazonaws.com/storage.citizensforethics.org/wp-content/uploads/2016/07/20022402/6-14-12_CREW_Letter_to_Aetna.pdf; "Top Organizations Disclosing Donations to American Action Network, 2018," Center for Responsive Politics, accessed March 1, 2020, https://www.opensecrets.org/outsidespending/contrib.php?cycle=2018&cmte=american%20action%20network.
14. Coalition Against Socialized Medicine website, accessed March 1, 2020, https://nosocializedmedicine.org.

Chapter 9

1. Marilyn Serafini, "Why Clinicians Support Single-Payer—and Who Will Win and Lose," *NEJM Catalyst* 4, no. 1 (2018).
2. Serafini, "Why Clinicians Support Single-Payer."
3. "Survey: 42% of Physicians Strongly Support Single Payer Healthcare, 35% Strongly Oppose," Merritt Hawkins, August 14, 2017, https://www.merritthawkins.com/uploadedFiles/mha_singlepayer_press_release_2017(1).pdf.
4. Roger Collier, "American Medical Association Membership Woes Continue," *Canadian Medical Association Journal* 183, no. 11 (August 9, 2011): E713–14, https://doi.org/10.1503/cmaj.109-3943.
5. "AMA Vision on Health Care Reform," American Medical Association, accessed February 16, 2020, https://www.ama-assn.org/delivering-care/patient-support-advocacy/ama-vision-health-care-reform.
6. Shannon Firth, "AMA President: It's Still 'No' to Single Payer," MedPage Today, October 17, 2018, https://www.medpagetoday.com/publichealthpolicy/healthpolicy/75775.
7. Dylan Scott, "The Nation's Most Prominent Doctors Group Almost Dropped Its Opposition to Medicare-for-All," Vox, June 12, 2019, https://www.vox.com/policy-and-politics/2019/6/12/18662722/ama-medicare-for-all-single-payer-vote-2020.

8. American College of Physicians, "Nation's Top Primary Care Physician Organizations Release Guidelines for Patient-Centered Medical Home Recognition Programs," accessed February 16, 2020, https://www.acponline.org/acp-newsroom/nations-top-primary-care-physician-organizations-releaseguidelines-for-patient-centered-medical-home.
9. Steffie Woolhandler and David U. Himmelstein, "Administrative Work Consumes One-Sixth of U.S. Physicians' Working Hours and Lowers Their Career Satisfaction," *International Journal of Health Services: Planning, Administration, Evaluation* 44, no. 4 (2014): 635–42, https://doi.org/10.2190/HS.44.4.a.
10. Brendan Murphy, "For First Time, Physician Practice Owners Are Not the Majority," American Medical Association, May 31, 2017, https://www.ama-assn.org/practice-management/economics/first-time-physician-practice-owners-are-not-majority.
11. Maggie Wade, "3 Miss. Doctors Say They Were Fired After Speaking Up About COVID-19 Safety," WMC Action News 5 (Memphis, TN), April 6, 2020, https://www.wmcactionnews5.com/2020/04/07/miss-doctors-say-they-were-fired-after-speaking-up-about-covid-safety.
12. Janet Adamy and Paul Overberg, "Doctors, Once GOP Stalwarts, Now More Likely to Be Democrats," *Wall Street Journal*, October 6, 2019, https://www.wsj.com/articles/doctors-once-gop-stalwarts-now-more-likely-to-be-democrats-11570383523.
13. Eric Lopez, Tricia Newman, Gretchen Jacobson, et al., "How Much More Than Medicare Do Private Insurers Pay? A Review of the Literature," Kaiser Family Foundation, April 15, 2020, https://www.kff.org/medicare/issue-brief/how-much-more-than-medicare-do-private-insurers-pay-a-review-of-the-literature/.
14. Ronen Avraham, Leemore S Dafny, and Max M. Schanzenbach, "The Impact of Tort Reform on Employer-Sponsored Health Insurance Premiums," *Journal of Law, Economics, and Organization* 28, no. 4 (2012): 657–86.
15. Sandra Levy and Leslie Kane, "MedScape Malpractice Report 2017," November 15, 2017, https://www.medscape.com/slideshow/2017-malpractice-report-6009206.
16. Clara Felice and Litsa Lambkros, "Medical Liability in Three Single-Payer Countries," PNHP, n.d.; Stephen Clarke, "Medical Malpractice Liability: Canada," Library of Congress Law Library,

June 2009, https://www.loc.gov/law/help/medical-malpractice-liability/canada.php.

17. Ken Budd, "7 Ways to Reduce Medical School Debt," Association of American Medical Colleges, October 9, 2018, https://www.aamc.org/news-insights/7-ways-reduce-medical-school-debt.
18. Julie P. Phillips et al., "A Retrospective Analysis of the Relationship Between Medical Student Debt and Primary Care Practice in the United States," *Annals of Family Medicine* 12, no. 6 (2014): 542–49.
19. Robert A. Dugger et al., "The Color of Debt: Racial Disparities in Anticipated Medical Student Debt in the United States," *PloS One* 8, no. 9 (2013).
20. Sara Nelson, "Solidarity Is a Force Stronger Than Gravity," *Jacobin*, August 2019, https://jacobinmag.com/2019/08/sara-nelson-afa-democratic-socialists-convention.
21. Michael Wayland, "GM Reinstates Health Insurance for Striking UAW Members," CNBC, September 26, 2019, https://www.cnbc.com/2019/09/26/gm-reinstates-health-insurance-for-striking-uaw-members.html.
22. "Organizations That Endorse H.R. 1384," Medicare for All Resolutions, accessed March 1, 2020, https://www.medicare4allresolutions.org/endorsing-organizations/.
23. Amanda Gomez, "Here's What Unions Think About Medicare for All," ThinkProgress, July 12, 2019, https://archive.thinkprogress.org/what-unions-think-about-medicare-for-all-2cffd87d7814.
24. Chelsea Janes, David Weigel, and Holly Bailey, "Sen. Bernie Sanders Changes How Medicare-for-All Plan Treats Union Contracts in Face of Opposition by Organized Labor," *Washington Post*, August 21, 2019, https://www.washingtonpost.com/politics/sen-bernie-sanders-changes-medicare-for-all-plan-in-face-of-opposition-by-organized-labor/2019/08/21/d8144e06-c423-11e9-9986-1fb3e4397be4_story.html.
25. Elizabeth Warren, "Ending the Stranglehold of Health Care Costs on American Families," n.d., https://elizabethwarren.com/plans/paying-for-m4a.
26. Donald Trump, "Democrats 'Medicare for All' Plan Will Demolish Promises to Seniors," *USA Today*, October 10, 2018, https://www.usatoday.com/story/opinion/2018/10/10/donald-trump-democrats-open-borders-medicare-all-single-payer-column/1560533002.

27. American Public Health Association, "Fact Sheet: Prescription Medication Use by Older Adults," Medscape, accessed February 16, 2020, http://www.medscape.com/viewarticle/501879.
28. US Department of Health and Human Services, "Costs of Care—Long-Term Care Information," October 10, 2017, https://longtermcare.acl.gov/costs-how-to-pay/costs-of-care.html.
29. Amber Willink, Cathy Shoen, and Karen Davis, "How Medicare Could Provide Dental, Vision, and Hearing Care for Beneficiaries," Issue Brief, Commonwealth Fund, January 2018, https://www.commonwealthfund.org/publications/issue-briefs/2018/jan/how-medicare-could-provide-dental-vision-and-hearing-care.
30. Lance Stevens and Lawrence Mallory, "U.S. Seniors Pay Billions, Yet Many Cannot Afford Healthcare," Gallup, April 15, 2019, https://news.gallup.com/opinion/gallup/248741/seniors-pay-billions-yet-cannot-afford-healthcare.aspx.
31. Michael Anne Kyle et al., "Financial Hardships of Medicare Beneficiaries with Serious Illness," *Health Affairs* 38, no. 11 (2019): 1801–6.
32. Steve Finlay, "GM Is Getting Sick of High Health-Care Costs," *Ward's Dealer Business* 38, no. 3 (2004): 22.
33. "Options to Finance Medicare for All," Office of Senator Sanders, n.d., https://www.sanders.senate.gov/download/options-to-finance-medicare-for-all?inline=file.
34. G. Claxton et al., "Employer Health Benefits: 2019 Annual Survey," Kaiser Family Foundation, 2019, http://files.kff.org/attachment/Report-Employer-Health-Benefits-Annual-Survey-2019.
35. Simon Johnson, Betsey Stevenson, and Mark Zandi, "Warren Medicare for All Plan Revenue Estimate Letter," October 31, 2019, https://assets.ctfassets.net/4ubxbgy9463z/27ao9rfB6MbQgGmaXK4eGc/d06d5a224665324432c6155199afe0bf/Medicare_for_All_Revenue_Letter___Appendix.pdf.
36. Claxton et al., "Employer Health Benefits: 2019 Annual Survey."
37. Christina Farr, "Apple Is Launching Medical Clinics to Deliver the 'World's Best Health Care Experience' to Its Employees," CNBC, February 27, 2018, https://www.cnbc.com/2018/02/27/apple-launching-medical-clinics-for-employees.html.
38. Corynne Cirilli, "The US Chamber of Commerce Might Not Be What You Think," Racked, October 2, 2017, https://www.racked.com/2017/10/2/16370014/us-chamber-commerce-explainer; "U.S. Chamber Letter to the Senate Opposing Medicare for All and

Medicare Buy-In Proposals," US Chamber of Commerce, March 18, 2019, https://www.uschamber.com/letter/us-chamber-letter-the-senate-opposing-medicare-all-and-medicare-buy-proposals.

39. "Top Spenders: 2019," Center for Responsive Politics, 2020, https://www.opensecrets.org/federal-lobbying/top-spenders?cycle=2019.
40. Rhett Buttle, Katie Wonnenberg, and Angela Simaan, "Small-Business Owners' Views on Health Coverage and Costs," Issue Brief, Commonwealth Fund, September 2019, https://www.commonwealthfund.org/publications/issue-briefs/2019/sep/small-business-owners-views-health-coverage-costs.
41. "United States Small Business Profile, 2019," Small Business Administration Office of Advocacy, 2019, https://cdn.advocacy.sba.gov/wp-content/uploads/2019/04/23142719/2019-Small-Business-Profiles-US.pdf; Elaine Pofeldt, "Million-Dollar, One-Person Business Revolution Accelerates," *Forbes*, June 27, 2019, https://www.forbes.com/sites/elainepofeldt/2019/06/27/million-dollar-one-person-business-revolution-accelerates; Buttle, Wonnenberg, and Simaan, "Small-Business Owners' Views on Health Coverage and Costs."
42. "United States Small Business Profile, 2019."
43. Physicians for a National Health Program, "Launch of 'Business for Medicare for All.' " https://pnhp.org/news/launch-of-business-for-medicare-for-all/; "Business Leaders for Health Care Transformation," https://www.blhct.org/

Chapter 10

1. Robert J. Blendon and John M. Benson, "Americans' Views on Health Policy: A Fifty-Year Historical Perspective," *Health Affairs* 20, no. 2 (2001): 33–46.
2. Kaiser Family Foundation, "Public Opinion on Single-Payer, National Health Plans, and Expanding Access to Medicare Coverage," May 27, 2020, https://www.kff.org/slideshow/public-opinion-on-single-payer-national-health-plans-and-expanding-access-to-medicare-coverage.
3. "About Us," Partnership for America's Health Care Future, https://americashealthcarefuture.org/about-us; "Americans Don't Want a One-Size-Fits-All Government Health Insurance System When They Learn the Facts," Partnership for America's Health Care Future, February 5, 2020, https://americashealthcarefuture.org/

americans-dont-want-a-one-size-fits-all-government-health-insurance-system-when-they-learn-the-facts; "ICYMI: One-Size-Fits-All Systems 'Don't Actually Put the Patient at the Center of Their Care, Don't Address Costs,'" Partnership for America's Health Care Future, February 6, 2020, https://americashealthcarefuture.org/icymi-one-size-fits-all-systems-dont-actually-put-the-patient-at-the-center-of-their-care-dont-address-costs.

4. Pew Research Center, "Attitudes on Same-Sex Marriage," May 14, 2019, https://www.pewforum.org/fact-sheet/changing-attitudes-on-gay-marriage.
5. David Cole, *Engines of Liberty: The Power of Citizen Activists to Make Constitutional Law* (Basic Books, 2016).
6. Ryan Grim, *We've Got People: From Jesse Jackson to AOC, the End of Big Money and the Rise of a Movement* (Strong Arm Press, 2019).
7. "Idaho Expand Medicaid Ballot Measure Results 2018," CNN, last updated December 21, 2018, https://www.cnn.com/election/2018/results/idaho/ballot-measures/1.
8. Pew Research Center, "The Partisan Divide on Political Values Grows Even Wider," October 5, 2017, https://www.people-press.org/2017/10/05/the-partisan-divide-on-political-values-grows-even-wider.
9. Pew Research Center, "The Partisan Divide on Political Values Grows Even Wider."
10. Kaiser Family Foundation, "Public Opinion on Single-Payer, National Health Plans, and Expanding Access to Medicare Coverage."
11. "About Us," Partnership for America's Health Care Future.
12. Lee Fang and Nick Surgey, "Lobbyist Documents Reveal Health Care Industry Battle Plan Against 'Medicare for All,'" The Intercept, November 20, 2018, https://theintercept.com/2018/11/20/medicare-for-all-healthcare-industry.
13. Adam Cancryn, "The Army Built to Fight 'Medicare for All,'" Politico, November 25, 2019, https://www.politico.com/news/agenda/2019/11/25/medicare-for-all-lobbying-072110.
14. Holly Otterbein and Maya King, "Anti-Medicare for All Ad Campaign Launches in South Carolina," Politico, February 26, 2020, https://www.politico.com/news/2020/02/26/anti-medicare-for-all-south-carolina-117771; David Weigel, "Signs of Change in Elizabeth Warren's Campaign," *Washington Post*, December 3, 2019, https://www.washingtonpost.com/politics/paloma/the-trailer/

2019/12/03/the-trailer-signs-of-change-in-elizabeth-warren-s-campaign/5de51e95602ff1181f2641f2.
15. "The Truth About One-Size-Fits-All Government Insurance Systems," Partnership for America's Health Care Future, 2019, https://americashealthcarefuture.org/risk.
16. Cancryn, "The Army Built to Fight 'Medicare for All.'"
17. "Industries," Center for Responsive Politics, 2019, https://www.opensecrets.org/federal-lobbying/industries?cycle=a.
18. "Fighting Voter Suppression," American Civil Liberties Union, 2016, https://www.aclu.org/issues/voting-rights/fighting-voter-suppression.

Chapter 11

1. Nouriel Roubini, "The Coming Greater Depression of the 2020s," Project Syndicate, April 28, 2020, https://www.project-syndicate.org/commentary/greater-depression-covid19-headwinds-by-nouriel-roubini-2020-04.

INDEX